Fundamentals of Electrocardiography and Vectorcardiography

Fundamentals of Electrocardiography and Vectorcardiography

By

LAWRENCE E. LAMB, M.D.

Director of Cardiology and
Chief, Department of Internal Medicine
Air University
School of Aviation Medicine, USAF
Randolph Air Force Base, Texas
Consultant in Cardiology
3700th USAF Hospital
Lackland Air Force Base
San Antonio, Texas

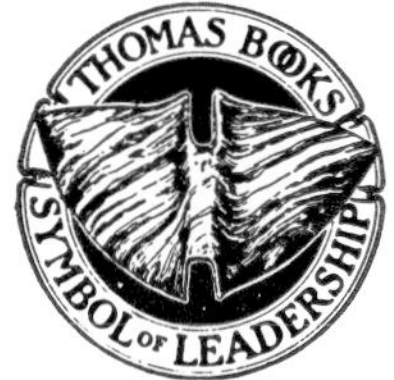

CHARLES C THOMAS · PUBLISHER
Springfield · Illinois · U.S.A.

CHARLES C THOMAS • PUBLISHER
BANNERSTONE HOUSE
301-327 East Lawrence Avenue, Springfield, Illinois, U.S.A.

Published simultaneously in the British Commonwealth of Nations by
BLACKWELL SCIENTIFIC PUBLICATIONS, LTD., OXFORD, ENGLAND

Published simultaneously in Canada by
THE RYERSON PRESS, TORONTO

Library of Congress Catalog Card Number: 57-6865

Printed in the United States of America

To My Friend and Teacher

Dr. Pierre W. Duchosal

Geneva, Switzerland

Preface

THE PURPOSE of this book is to set forth the basic fundamentals of electrocardiography and vectorcardiography. The rapid growth of this important field behooves a clear understanding of the principles involved. It is no longer sufficient to memorize patterns, or for that matter to memorize a group of rules incorporated under the term vector electrocardiography. The reader should learn from the beginning the laws governing the measurement of potential from the surface of a volume conductor, the effects of eccentricity of the heart, the effects of lead length on measurements, and the very definite limitations of many of the instruments currently employed (direct writing instrument in particular). He should learn the fundamentals of vector analysis as a mathematical science, e.g., unless one understands the fundamental difference between polygons and coordinate graphs there is not much probability of comprehending the difference between vectorcardiograms and electrocardiograms, or their similarities.

The manuscript begins at the very beginning with the simplest of vector concepts. More detailed or technical points are placed as footnotes for the more exacting reader and to avoid confusing the beginner. An abundant group of illustrations are used to clarify the text and to help the reader develop a three dimensional concept. Spatial models of vectorcardiograms are used as a further aid in grasping the spatial orientation of the electrical forces.

The emphasis on the mean spatial QRS-T angle in recent years has made it desirable for the practitioner to be able to determine this angle from the routing 12 lead electrocardiogram. For this purpose a simple chart is provided that may be used like an ordinary road mileage chart without resorting to cumbersome calculations.

The text includes the most modern concepts of cellular activity as well as reference to important basic experiments and concepts too soon forgotten. It is intended as a simplified book for the beginner as well as detailed footnotes and new concepts for the authority. The material points up the value of European concepts of electrical moment, not commonly employed by American cardiologists. A large number of authentic clinical illustrations are included to provide practical application.

L.E.L.

Acknowledgments

I WISH TO TAKE this opportunity to thank the following people who have helped to make this book possible. In particular I wish to thank Colonel Archie A. Hoffman for constructive suggestions, Dr. Julian Ward for calculating the Vectorcardiogram Standardization Charts included in the appendix, and Dr. M. B. Danford and Mr. Richard McNee of the Department of Biometrics for performing the calculations for the Spatial Angle Chart. I am especially pleased with the drawing of the illustrations done by Mr. Leonard F. Carol and assistants. The work done by technicians, Sara Johnson, Harvey Hamel, William Yarwood and Robert Wanner, in preparing the electrocardiograms and the vectorcardiogram models was an important contribution. I am indebted to Hedwig Richter and Patricia Dyer for the tedious job of typing the manuscript. The photography was done by Captain Arthur Thiesen, Sergeant Harvey Kohnitz and staff. To all of these people and the numerous other members of the staff of the School of Aviation Medicine that have helped, I wish to say thank you.

L.E.L.

Contents

Fundamentals of Electrocardiography and Vectorcardiography

I

Fundamental Vector Concepts

ELECTROCARDIOGRAPHY strives to measure potential (forces) created by the heart in terms of magnitude, direction and duration of action. Vector concepts greatly simplify analysis of these forces. The use of vectors to express mathematical quantities is as old as mathematics itself. They were applied to electrocardiography by Einthoven. The understanding of electrocardiography begins with an understanding of simple vector principles.

What Is a Vector? It is a symbol used to describe the characteristics of a force. The magnitude of the force is represented by the length of the vector. The arrow head (terminus) of the vector indicates the direction of the force. A vector used to describe a force in two dimensions (flat surface) is drawn as a flat arrow. A spatial vector representation is used to describe a three dimensional force (Fig. 1). The duration of action of a force is not expressed by a

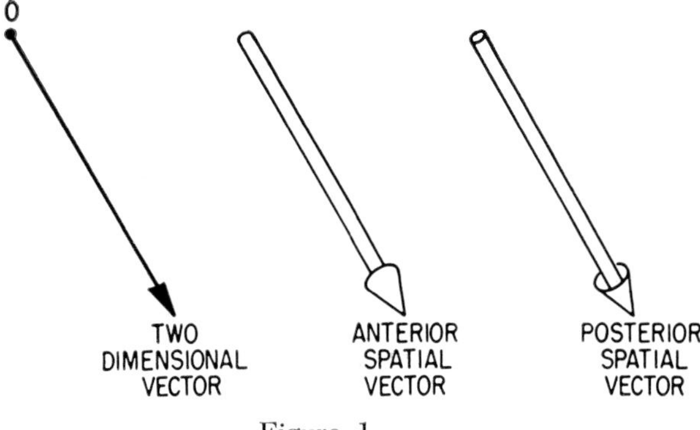

Figure 1.

vector unless the magnitude has been converted to time units. A force of one dyne acting for ten sec. is still a one dyne force represented by one unit length (1 unit equals 1 dyne). Expressed in time units as dynes × seconds, such a force would be equal to ten dyne seconds and represented by ten units length (1 unit equals 1 dyne second).

What Is the Point of Origin? The maximum effect of a force occurs at a point. The force is said to act on this point. In vector terminology this point is called the point of origin. One end of any vector is its point of origin and the other end is the head (terminus) indicating the direction of the vector and extent of its magnitude.

What Is an Instantaneous Vector? A vector without duration of time is an instantaneous vector. It acts only at a point in time. In electrocardiography it is often of interest to speak of a vector acting at one particular time interval, thus the vector acting momentarily at .04 sec. after the onset of an event is spoken of as the .04 sec. vector. Such a vector is an instantaneous vector and acts only at that time interval. At .05 sec. after the onset of the same event the vector might be entirely different in magnitude and direction. The .05 vector would be another instantaneous vector.

What Is a Resultant Vector? When two or more vectors are acting on a common point of origin, their net effect can be represented by a single vector. Such a vector is called a resultant vector (Fig. 2). It represents the effective force of all the vectors. *The resultant vector is not equal to the magnitude of all the vectors acting on the point, nor does it have a consistent relationship to their magnitude.*

What Is a Coordinate? Any straight line drawn through the point of origin is a coordi-

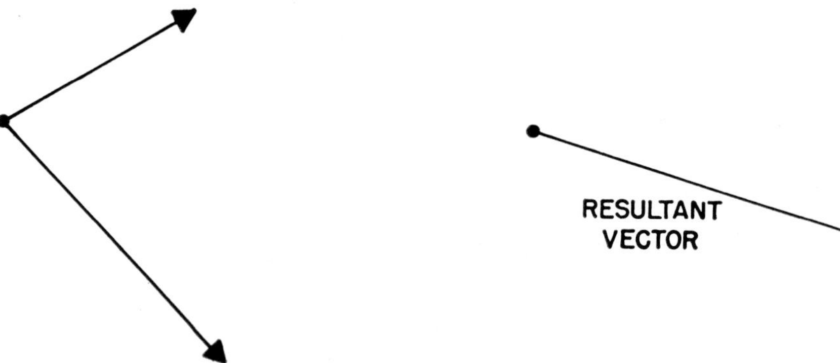

Figure 2.

nate. Its length can be marked off into units of measure. The effect of a vector in the direction defined by the coordinate (line) can be determined by constructing a perpendicular from the coordinate to the tip of the vector (Fig. 3). The units along the coordinate equals the effect of

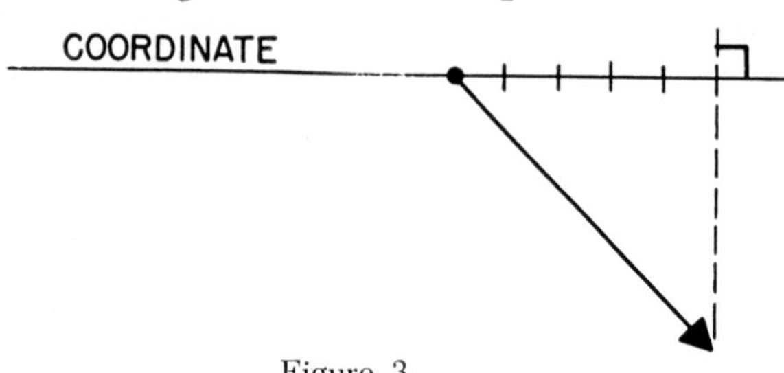

Figure 3.

the vector in that direction. This value is the coordinate value of the vector. The value may be expressed as positive or minus units by designating one end of the coordinate positive and the other negative.

The coordinate value of the vector is spoken of as its projection upon the coordinate. All electrocardiographic leads are coordinates and measure forces that are projected upon them. Any vector can be described in terms of its projection upon three mutually perpendicular coordinates (X, Y, Z). The X coordinate (transverse) defines the left to right location of the terminus. The Y coordinate (vertical) defines the vector terminus above or below the point of origin. The Z coordinate (sagittal) locates the vector terminus anterior or posterior to the point of origin (Fig. 4).

What Are Component Vectors? The units of magnitude measured upon the coordinates X, Y,

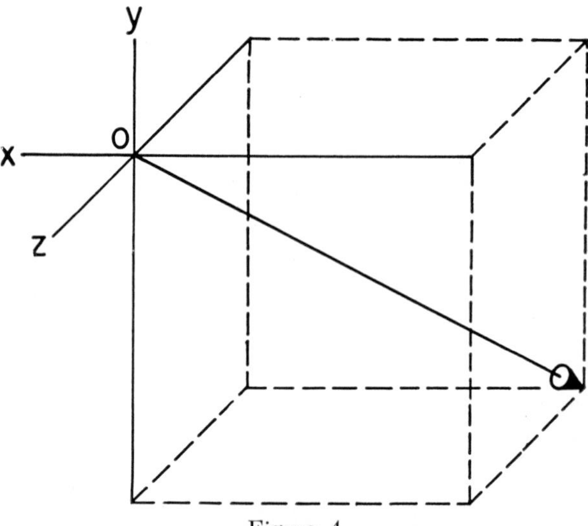

Figure 4.

Z can be expressed as vectors. The three vectors, X, Y, Z, are component vectors. The resultant of three such vector components is equal to the magnitude and direction of the spatial vector. They are perpendicular vector components (Fig. 5). Any spatial vector can be resolved into its three perpendicular components. The magnitude of the spatial vector can be calculated from its perpendicular components from the simple formula:

$$(\text{Spatial vector})^2 = X^2 + Y^2 + Z^2.$$

Any spatial vector may have multiple component vectors and multiple coordinates but it can have only three mutually perpendicular coordinates and three mutually perpendicular components.

How Is the Coordinate Value of a Vector Calculated? When the angle between a vector and a given coordinate is known the projection

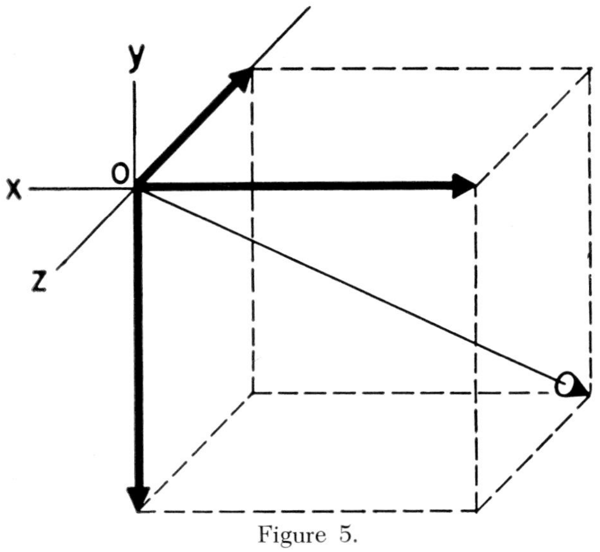

Figure 5.

of the vector on the coordinate can be calculated without constructing a perpendicular (Fig. 6). This is done by using the principle of the right triangle. The vector is the hypotenuse of a right triangle and the coordinate is the adjacent side. The cosine* of the angle times the magnitude of the vector equals its coordinate value:

$$\text{Cos} \propto \times \text{Vector Magnitude} = \text{Coordinate Value.}$$

*The cosine of an angle is equal to adjacent side divided by the hypotenuse.

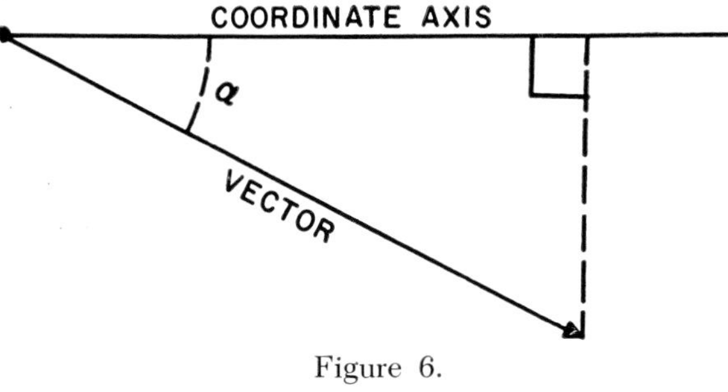

Figure 6.

What Is a Plane? A plane expresses two dimensions of a vector and has two perpendicular coordinates. It is a flat surface. *The frontal plane* (X, Y) is made up of the X, Y coordinates. *The transverse plane* (X, Z) is composed of the X, Z coordinates. *The sagittal plane* (Z, Y) is the Z, Y coordinates. These planes are mutually perpendicular to each other. Any two of them can be used to determine a spatial vector as two perpendicular planes include all three mutually perpendicular coordinates (X, Y, Z).

The principle of measuring a vector from its projection upon a plane or flat surface is frequently used in electrocardiography. The magnitude of a vector measured by a plane diminishes as the vector is rotated away from its flat surface (Fig. 7). Considering the frontal plane, as the vector is rotated away from the X, Y coordinates the frontal plane vector becomes smaller. Finally, when the vector is parallel to the Z coordinate its entire magnitude is measured by the Z coordinate. Such a vector has no projection upon the X or Y coordinate and has no magnitude value in the frontal plane. Both X and Y are perpendicular to Z and the frontal plane is perpendicular to such a vector. A simple rule is illustrated, *there is no force at any point on a plane perpendicular to a vector.* The direction of a vector can be determined by locating its perpendicular plane as the vector is 90° away from this plane.

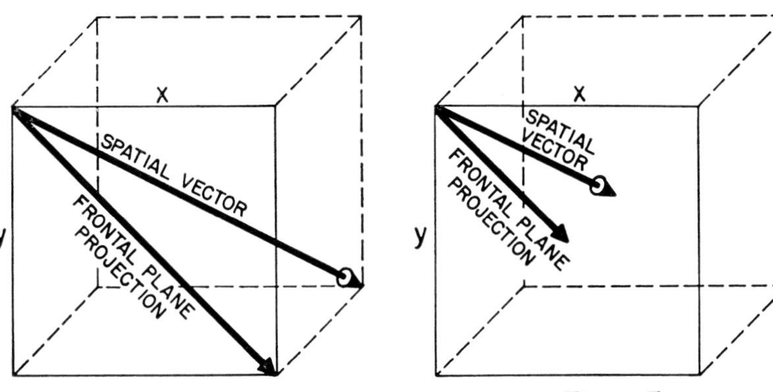

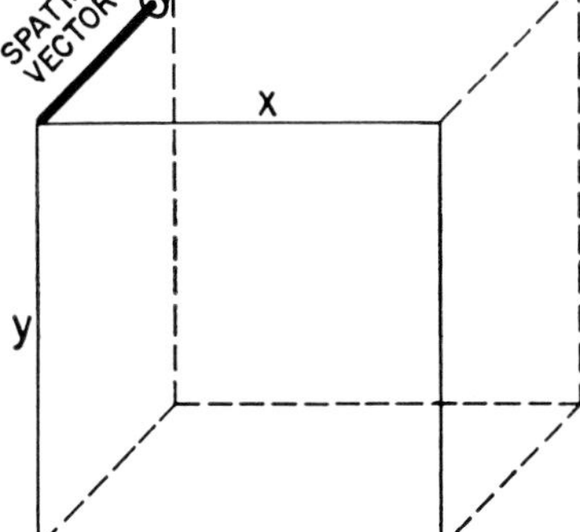

Figure 7.

What Is the Law of Parallelograms? The resultant of two vectors acting upon a common point can be determined by constructing a parallelogram (Fig. 8). The two vectors are two adjacent sides (a, b) of the parallelogram. The diagonal of the parallelogram is the resultant vector (c). The magnitude of the vectors act-

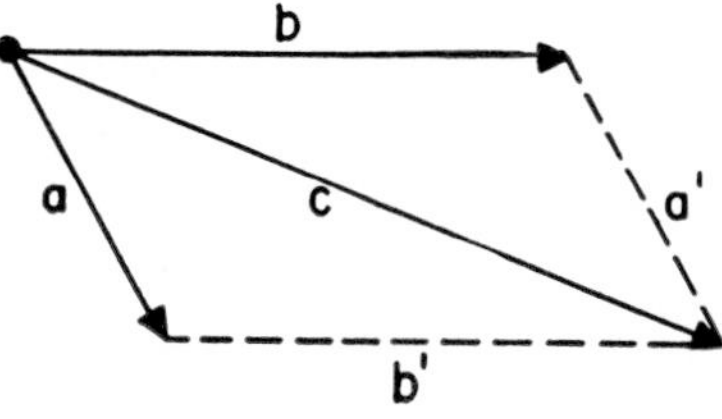

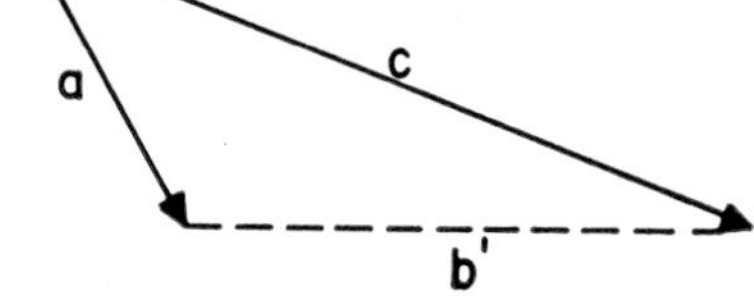

Figure 8.

ing on the common point can be determined from the sides of the parallelogram (a, b'). Note that $b = b'$ as they are opposite sides of the parallelogram. Knowing only a and c the magnitude of the vector b can be determined by merely measuring the distance between vector a and c or the length of b'. The two adjacent sides of the parallelogram equals the magnitude of the acting vectors and the diagonal equals their effect or resultant.

It is very important to realize that the diagonal of the parallelogram is not equivalent to the magnitude of the acting vectors. Any triangle is a semiparallelogram. When one side of a triangle is a component (acting) vector (a) and the other the resultant vector (c) the other component vector (b) can be determined from the law of parallelograms.

The Law of Simple Consecutive Vector Addition. The addition of vectors upon a common point, one after another, will cause the resultant vector to change with the addition of each vector. Consider eight vectors of equal magnitude (P) consecutively added to each other upon a common point (O) and directed 45° away from each other (Fig. 9). The addition of vector 2 to vector 1 creates the resultant 1. Note that R_1 is the diagonal of a semiparallelogram while V1 and V2 are the adjacent sides of the parallelogram. The addition of vector 3 to vectors 1 and 2 creates the resultant vector 2.

The addition of each new vector causes the resultant vector to rotate a distance equal to the added vector's magnitude. The rotating resultant vector describes an external pathway, comprised of the sides of a polygon. The length of the sides of the polygon is equal to the total magnitude of all the vectors acting on the common point. In this instance the magnitude of the eight vectors acting on the common point is 8P. The sum of the length of the sides of the polygon is also 8P. The graph of the rotating resultant vectors is a polygon. The resultants

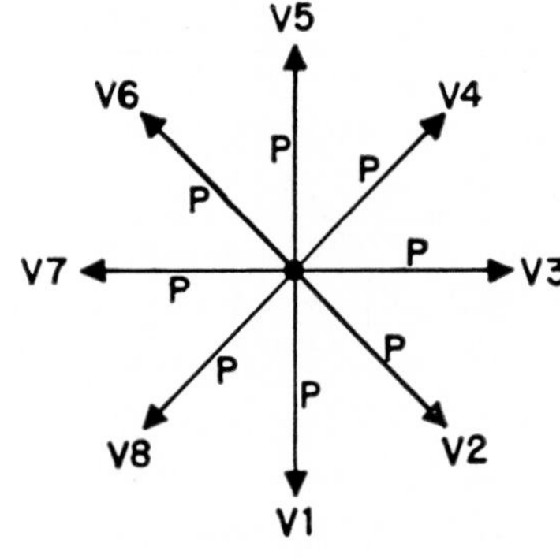

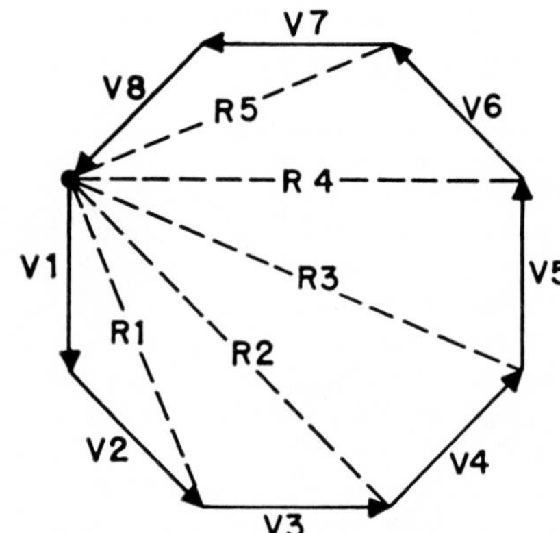

Figure 9.

originating from the center of origin may be called central resultants. Note that the magnitude of the acting vectors is never equal to the central resultants. A law may be formulated: *The consecutive addition of vectors upon a common point will cause the central resultant to rotate, describing a polygon. The length of the sides of the polygon is equal to the magnitude of the vectors added to each other.**

The Law of Simple Consecutive Vector Subtraction. The subtraction of vector forces, one after another, from a common point creates a similar situation as consecutive addition. Given eight vectors of equal magnitude (P) directed 45° away from each other, there will be no effective force until subtraction begins. With the subtraction of vector 1 an effective force is created by the remaining seven vectors. The subtraction of vector 2 changes the resultant again. The resultant vector changes with each additional subtraction. A law may be formulated: *The successive subtraction of vectors from a common point causes a resultant vector to be rotated describing a polygon. The length of the sides of the polygon is equal to the magnitude of the vectors subtracted.* In either addition or subtraction the shape of the polygon will also depend upon the order of addition or subtraction (Fig. 10).

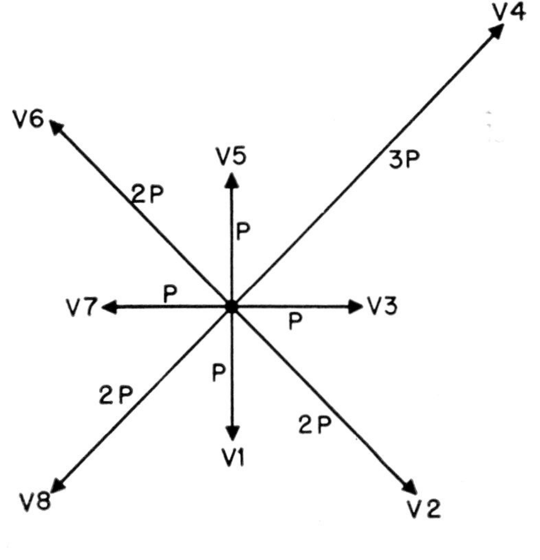

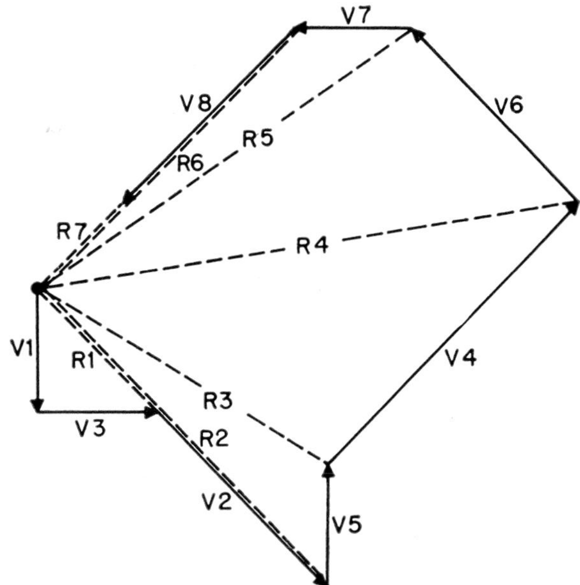

Figure 10. The irregular shaped polygon is created by unequal vectors acting upon the point of origin. Note that the simultaneous action of such unequal vectors would have a resultant, in this case R7. The resultant of several vectors acting on a common point can always be determined in this manner. In the previous illustrations the resultant has been zero and the polygon was a closed polygon.

The Law of Multiple Simultaneous Vector Addition. The addition of vectors upon a common point may be complicated by the simultaneous addition of more than one vector. Consider two vectors *a* and *b* added simultaneously to a previously existing vector, A (Fig. 11). Vectors *a* and *b* have a resultant effect, *c*, the diagonal of a parallelogram. The action of these two vectors is equal to vector *c*. When vectors

---

*Figure 9 is drawn to scale as geometric proof of the law. The method of polygon formation must apply to every situation wherein vectors are assumed to act upon a common point or center. The polygon finds its origin in the law of parallelograms. Whenever instantaneous resultant vectors are assumed to act on a point the sides of a polygon can be constructed. The sides of the polygon then represent the magnitude of the component vectors. The reader is referred to: White, Harvey E.: *Classical and Modern Physics.* New York, Van Nostrand Company, Inc., 1940, pp. 25-26, and Kimball, A. L.: *A College Text-Book of Physics,* Fifth Edition, New York, Henry Holt and Company, 1939, p. 11.

a and *b* are added to vector *A* it is exactly the same as if vector *c* had been added to vector *A*. Knowing vector *A* and the new resultant (*B*) created by the addition of vector *c*, one can determine vector *c* by measuring the distance between *A* and *B*. A law may be formulated: *The simultaneous addition of two or more vectors to a previously existing vector will cause it to rotate describing one side of a polygon. The length of the side is equal to the magnitude of the resultant of the simultaneously added vectors.* A similar relationship exists for subtraction.

What Is a Coordinate Graph? Electrocardiographic leads are coordinate graphs in contradistinction to vectorcardiograms which are polygons. They are vectors graphed upon a coordinate in a linear fashion. Extend coordinates X and Y through the circular type graph of consecutive vector addition (Fig. 12). Each central resultant can be projected upon the coordinates in a linear fashion. This creates a coordinate graph of the x components of central resultants and another graph of the y components of the central resultants. Note that such graphs are graphs of the central resultants and not the sides of the polygon. As shown above the magnitude of vectors acting on a common point is measured by the sides of a polygon. By indirect calculation or geometric construction the polygon can be obtained from linear coordinate graphs, but such a procedure must be carried out before one can speak correctly in terms of vector magnitude.*

What Is an Absolute Linear Graph? The central resultants may be graphed upon a time base to form a linear graph (Fig. 13). A popular application to vectorcardiography is to so graph the instantaneous resultant spatial vectors. It is clear from a fundamental vector approach that such central resultants in no way represent the magnitude of the component vectors acting upon a common point and unless one knows the angles between such central resultants the sides of the polygon cannot be reconstructed. These measurements have been called the absolute vectorcardiogram. A linear graph of the central resultants is called an absolute graph. Actually the use of the term absolute is a misnomer in

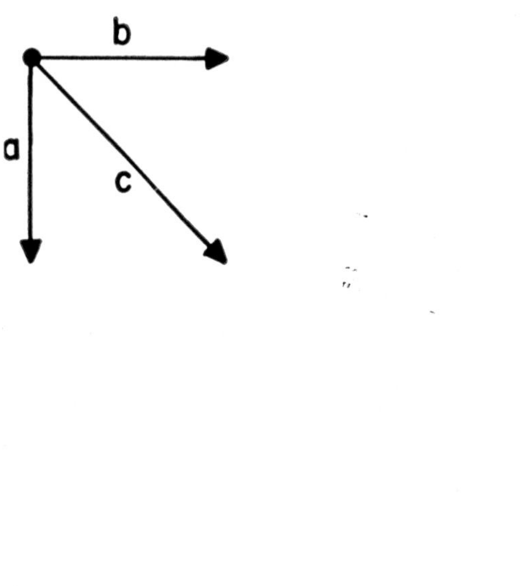

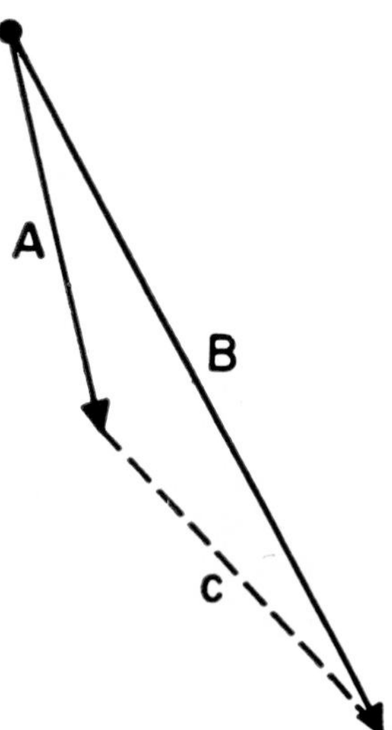

Figure 11.

*Each side of the polygon can be determined by obtaining its x and y component. The x component is the difference in amplitude of the central resultant projection upon x coordinate for that time interval and the y component is the difference in amplitude of the central resultant projected upon the y coordinate. The side for this time interval or for the added vector is then obtained from the formula $x^2 + y^2 = \text{Side}^2$ or by simple graphic construction.

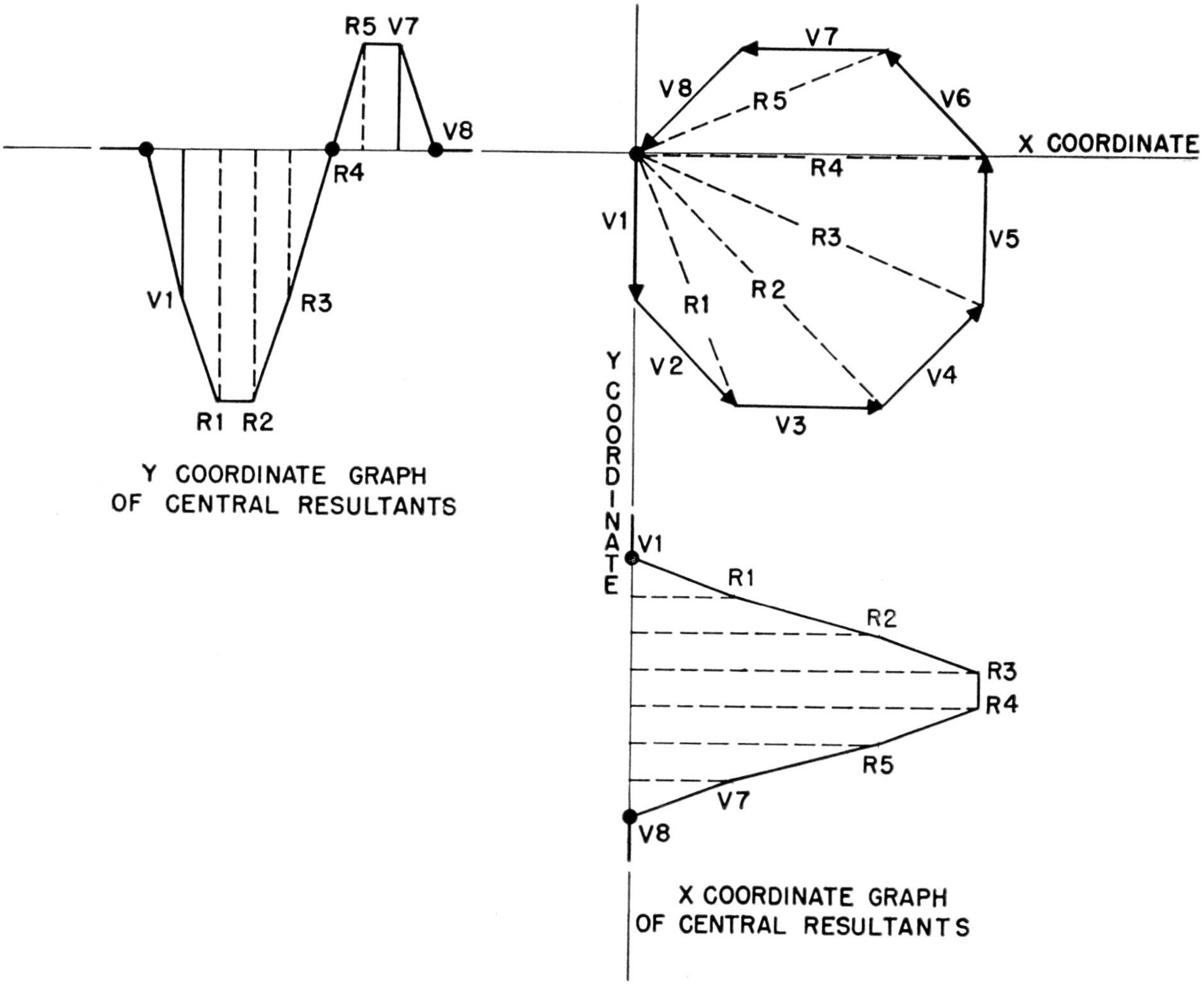

R5 V7
V8
R4
V1
R3
R1 R2
Y COORDINATE GRAPH
OF CENTRAL RESULTANTS
V7
V8
R5
V6
X COORDINATE
R4
V1
R3
V5
R1
R2
Y COORDINATE
V2
V4
V3
V1
R1
R2
R3
R4
R5
V7
V8
X COORDINATE GRAPH
OF CENTRAL RESULTANTS

Figure 12.

R5
R4
R3
R1
R2
R1 R2 R3 R4 R5

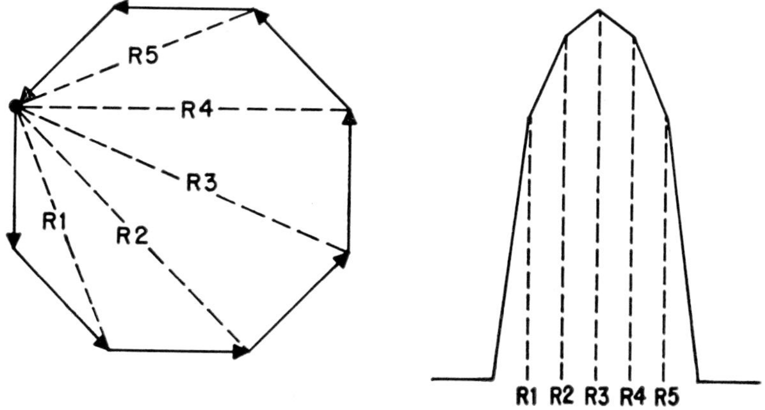

Figure 13.

that resultant vectors are not absolute measurements and such measurements of absolute quantities must be approached from the polygon principle.

Two different polygons can be constructed with entirely different length of sides and identical central resultants (Fig. 14). Even though the central resultants are the same the component vectors are not at all the same. This simple illustration demonstrates the fallacy of using instantaneous resultant vectors to measure magnitude of component vectors.

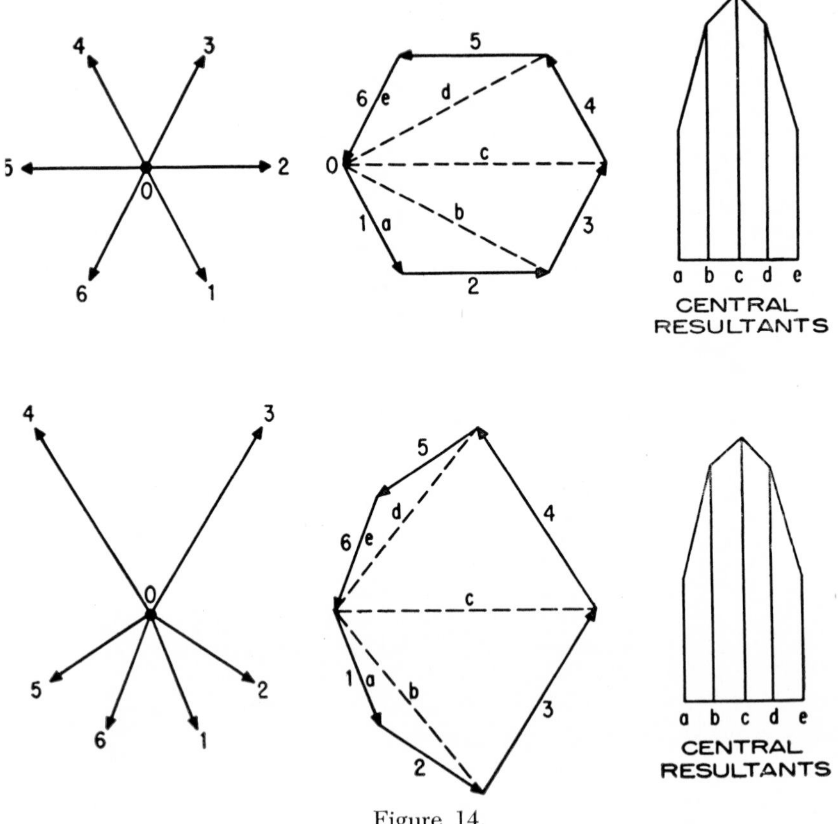

Figure 14.

Expression of Vector Magnitude In Time Units. Once the magnitude of a force is known it can be converted to units of time by multiplying its magnitude by its duration of action. When we are concerned with forces acting about a point the magnitude factor is obtained from the sides of the polygon. Consider a force of three dynes (*a*) acting upon a point (Fig. 15). Five seconds later a force is subtracted from the same point (*o*) creating a new resultant (*b*). The magnitude of the force subtracted is equal to the distance between the two resultants (*a* and *b*). If this distance is equivalent to a force of two dynes and its duration of action was five seconds, it can be expressed as ten dyne seconds (2 dynes × 5 sec.).

The "Mean" Vector from the Area of Coordinate Graphs. A popular concept in electro-

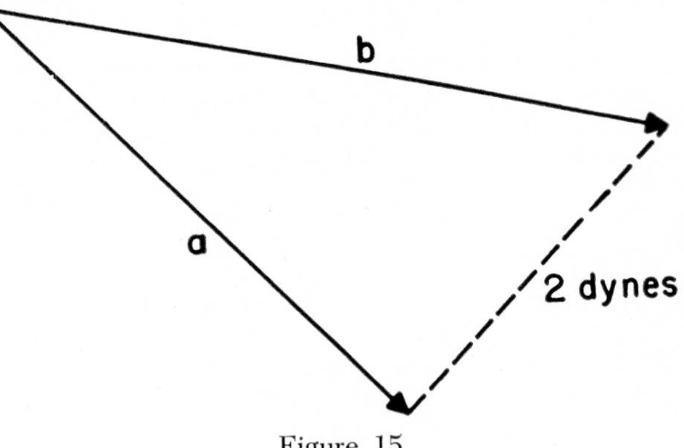

Figure 15.

cardiography is to obtain the "mean" vector (mean QRS or T) from calculations based on coordinate graphs (the leads themselves). The first step is to obtain the triangular area enclosed on a given coordinate.* This is the coordinate value for the "mean" vector. Another coordinate value is then obtained in a similar manner. A perpendicular is then constructed

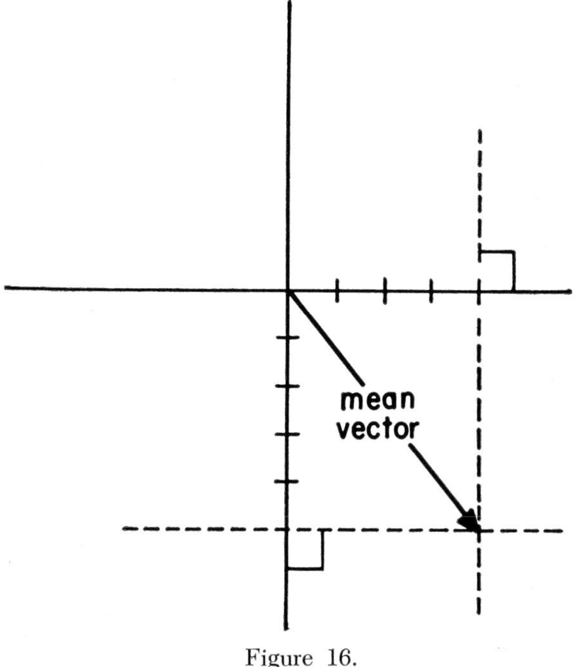

Figure 16.

to each of the two coordinates marking off their unit values. The point of intersection between the two perpendiculars is the terminus or the "mean" vector. The magnitude of the vector is depicted by its length and its direction by its axis and terminus (Fig. 16).

*The base of the triangle is a function of time and the amplitude of the complex is a function of magnitude. The height times the base divided by two is the triangular area. In the event that a triangular area exists above the coordinate it is positive and if below it is negative. If part of the coordinate graph has a positive value and the other part negative the two triangular areas are subtracted from each other or added by algebraic addition. This value represents the mean value measured by such a coordinate.

The term "mean" vector as determined by the above method is a misnomer. The vector magnitude has no consistent relationship to the magnitude of vectors acting about a common point. The basic premise for magnitude is in error as magnitude must first be determined from the polygon principle and then converted to time units. Nevertheless such graphs are satisfactory for determining the direction of the resultant vector created by multiple forces acting about a point.

Instantaneous Vector Versus Polygon Sides. A simple graphic demonstration of the difference in values obtained from instantaneous resultant vectors and the polygon is exemplified by travel. Driving by car from San Antonio to Houston to Dallas one describes two sides of a polygon. The actual road mileage is the sides of the polygon and can be equated to the work performance of the auto. The air mileage from San Antonio to Dallas is the resultant or instantaneous vector, being the resultant of the sides of the polygon. Obviously one cannot equate work done by the auto to the air mileage nor can any function derived from the air mileage alone be expected to represent the auto's true activity (Fig. 17).

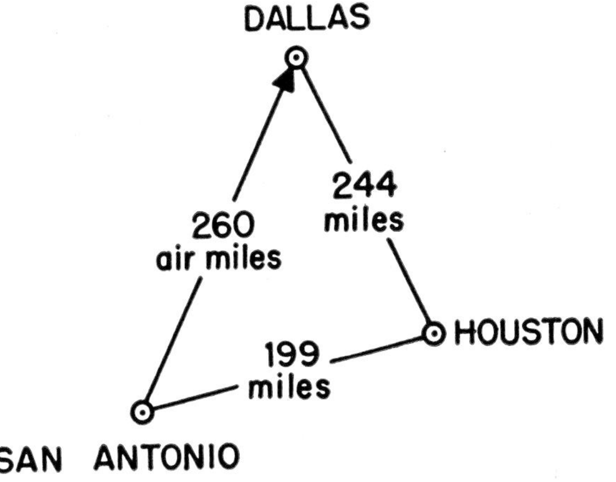

Figure 17.

II

Fundamental Cellular Concepts

THE ELECTRICAL EVENTS of the heart conform to basic principles of electrical physics. The events concern themselves with particles containing electrical energy. This, in turn, is related to the atomic structure of the elements or electrolytes found in the tissue mass and surrounding media. An intelligent understanding of the cell as a source of electrical activity requires at least a handshaking acquaintance with the fundamental behavior of particles bearing electrical energy.

THE CHARGED PARTICLE

Any particle containing electrical energy is a charged particle. Under proper environmental conditions this particle exerts a force. The magnitude of the force created by a particle is called its potential.* All charged particles are surrounded by an electrical field. The field is created by the transmission of potential into the surrounding media. Any point in this field has a potential value. The potential decreases at greater distances from the particle in accordance with the characteristics of the surrounding media. Since its potential is transmitted in all directions, the particle has no effective electrical force, i.e., the resultant force is zero (Fig. 18).

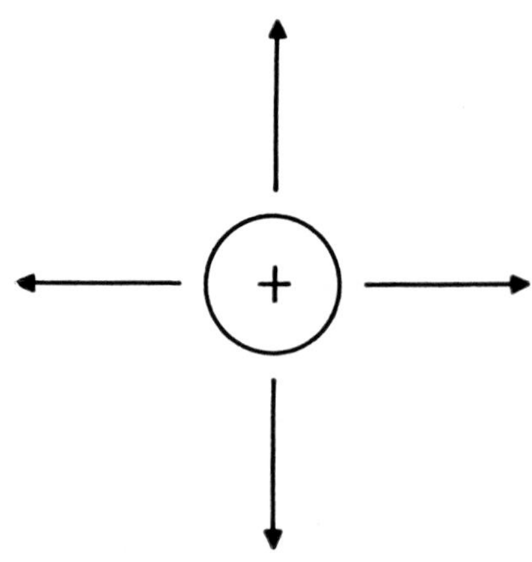

Figure 18.

THE DOUBLET

An effective electrical force or resultant force is created when two charged particles of different potential values are close enough to each other for overlapping of their electrical fields (Fig. 19). The force has direction and magnitude. The magnitude is equal to the difference in potential between the two particles. Potential difference is expressed in practical units as voltage. By convention, the particle of lesser charge is called negative and the particle of

*Potential is correctly defined as work. A unit of potential, one volt, is equal to 1/300 electrostatic unit, or 1/300 statvolt. An electrostatic unit difference in potential between two points exists when one erg of work is done to move one stat coulomb of positive charge from the point of least potential to the point of more positive potential. One erg is one dyne cm. or a force of one dyne acting a distance of one cm. Thus potential difference can be expressed in dyne cm. A dyne is a fundamental unit of force and is correctly given the dimension of magnitude.

Potential at a point is also expressed as work. The difference in potential is expressed between the point in question and earth potential, the latter being designated as zero potential.

Potential depends upon the charge that a particle bears, but is an expression of force not charge. Charge refers to the number of electrons contained by the particle. Current, expressed in amperes, is the amount of charge (coulombs) flowing per second. For further detail the reader is referred to: Gilbert, Norman E.: *Electricity and Magnetism*, Third Edition. New York, The Macmillan Company, 1950.

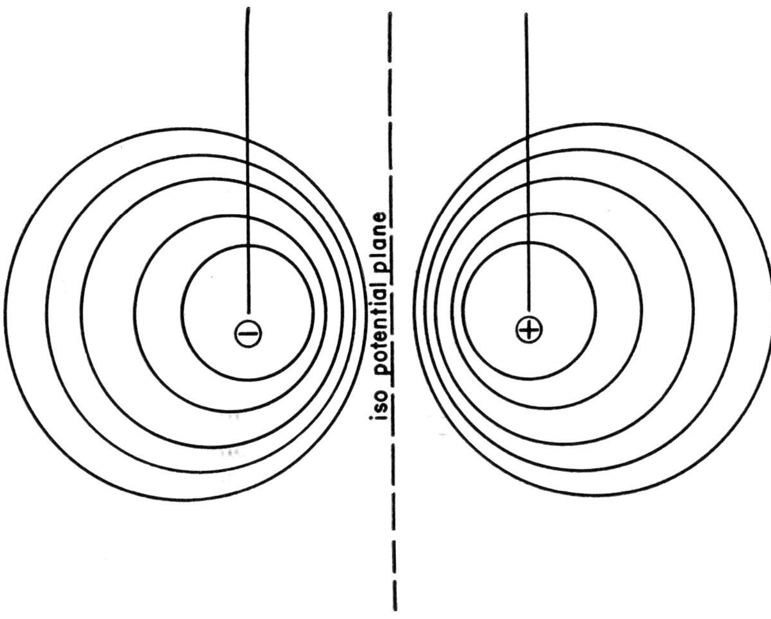

Figure 19.

greater charge, positive.* The electrical field surrounding the particle of greatest potential is called the positive electrical field and the field surrounding the point of least potential is called the negative electrical field. Between the two particles a zone must exist which is as positive to the negative particle as it is negative to the positive particle. This zone is created by the overlapping of the two electrical fields. The forces emitted from each particle tend to neutralize each other in the area between the two particles. This plane of neutralization is called the isoelectric or *isopotential plane.*

On the outer side of the positive particle the potential forces are unopposed and, of course, larger than those on the outer side of the negative particle. This difference in potential value creates a force directed away from the isopotential plane and toward the positive field. The maximum line of force must be in line with the axis between the positive and negative particles.

Such a line is perpendicular to the isopotential plane. The force acts as if it acted on a point where the line of force intersects the isopotential plane. This point is called the *"zero center."* It should be noted that this does not mean there is no potential at that point. It is a point of electrical neutrality. The force created by the electrical fields behaves as if it acted upon this point. The term *"zero center"* is an electrical term.

Two particles of different potential as described above create a force which may be described as a vector (Fig. 20). Its point of origin

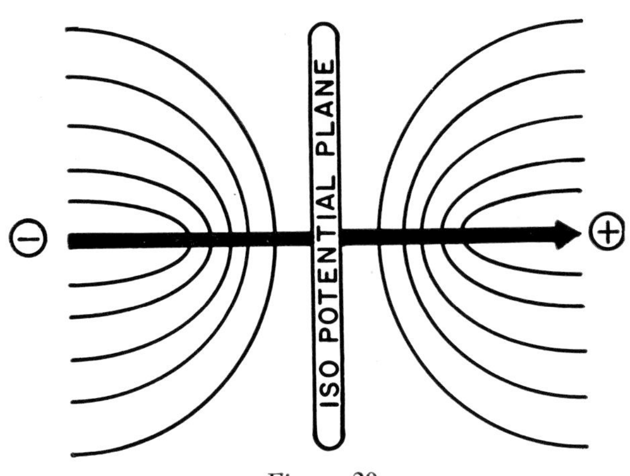

Figure 20.

*A particle may have less than zero potential in relation to earth potential. A particle may have negative potential in relation to another particle. As an illustration, if one particle has 35 units of potential and the other 5 units, the potential difference is 30 units. It is of no consequence where the zero point is placed. One may express their relative values as −15 and +15 with the same mathematical relationship.

is the zero center and its direction is toward the positive electrical field. The vector magnitude depends upon the difference in potential between the particles, their distance apart, and the character of the surrounding media. Two such particles are called a "*doublet.*" The force created by the doublet is called the *doublet vector.*

THE RESTING MUSCLE FIBER

The electrolytic content of the normal resting muscle fiber differs from the electrolytic content of its normal external environment. Consequently, there is a continuous diffusion of ions across the cell membrane. There is a natural tendency for ions to migrate from a location of higher density to one of lower density, thereby reaching a state of equilibrium. The difference in ionic concentration on either side of the membrane is the driving force of migration. The ionic activity may be altered by environmental factors. The diffusion of ions across the cell membrane also depends upon the character of the membrane itself. In this sense the membrane acts as a filter (dielectric constant) regulating the rate of diffusion between the two areas of different ionic content.

The diffusion of ions across the membrane and the character of the membrane filter are relatively stable in the normal resting state, thus creating a state of dynamic equilibrium. The external environment of the cell is relatively positive with respect to the internal environment (Fig. 21). A positive electrical field surrounds the muscle fiber. Thus, forces are directed externally at all points across the cell membrane. It is as if electrical doublets existed at all points around the cell. The resultant force is zero and *the resting cell creates no effective force in its surrounding media.* However, a force does exist across the cell membrane because the internal environment is negative with respect to the external environment. This potential difference is the *resting membrane action potential.* Experimental measurements have shown it to have a value of 50 to 90 mv.

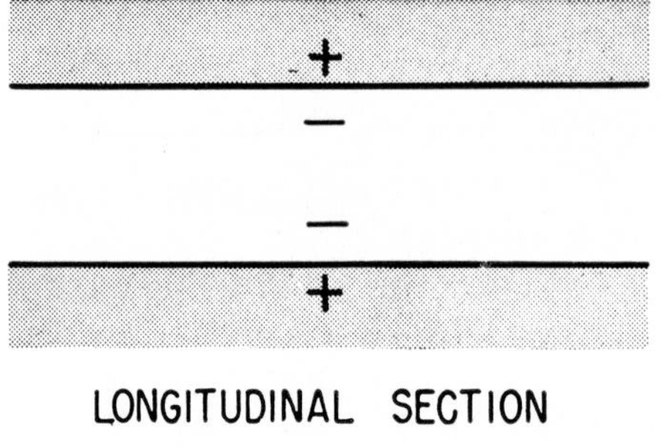

LONGITUDINAL SECTION

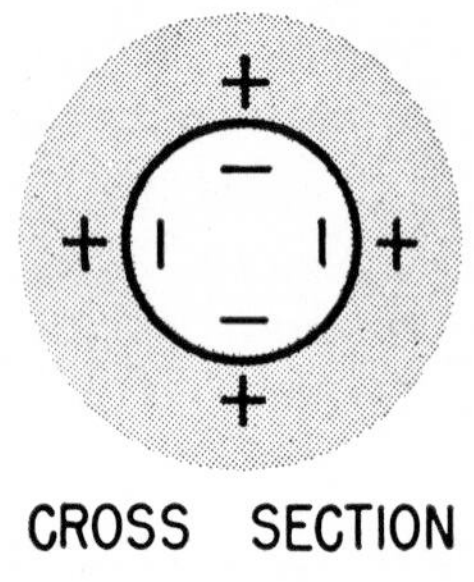

CROSS SECTION

RESTING MUSCLE FIBER

Figure 21.

EXCITATION

When the muscle fiber is stimulated a change occurs in the cell membrane. Stimulation may be accomplished by mechanical, chemical or electrical means. The membrane potential is altered and its behavior as a filter is changed. This permits a change in dynamic diffusion of electrolytes across the membrane. The initial event is the migration of sodium ions from the external environment to the internal environment, or an inward current of sodium. Stimulation increases the permeability of the cell membrane to sodium and, since there is a higher concentration of sodium externally, sodium migrates inward.

The change in the potential of the membrane and the change in electrolytic content of the internal and external cellular environment creates a positive electrical field within the cell with respect to its external environment (negative field). One may call this a reversal of the membrane action potential. The area of the muscle fiber which has undergone this change is said to be in the *"excited state."* The force created by the difference in potential is directed inward from all external points, perpendicular to the cell membrane. The resultant force is zero and there is no effective force in the external media distant to the cell. A rule may be formulated: *An area of muscle in the excited state creates no effective force in its surrounding media.*

During excitation of a muscle fiber there must exist an area in the excited state and an area in the resting state. At the junction of these two areas the active process of excitation is occurring. This boundary is *the wave of excitation* (Fig. 22). As pointed out above, neither the area in the excited nor resting state creates a force in the surrounding media. The force created at any instant in the external media is due to the boundary between muscle areas in different electrical states, in this case, the wave of excitation. Such a force is created at the surface of the cell and not across the cell membrane.*

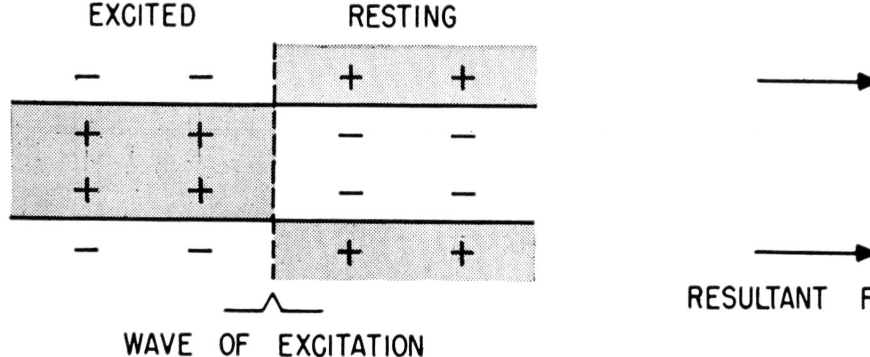

Figure 22.

*The force parallel to the surface may be explained by considering the field created perpendicular to flowing current as in the Oersted experiment. The wave front defines the border between current flowing in two different directions. The bidirectional current creates a force perpendicular to the direction of current flow, and perpendicular to the wave front.

RECOVERY

After completion of excitation the characteristics of the cell membrane as a filter are such that its permeability to potassium ions is increased. Since there is a larger concentration of potassium within the cell, potassium ions migrate outward, creating an outward current of potassium. The migration of potassium continues until a critical level is reached in the difference between intra and extracellular concentration. At this point the cell membrane completes recovery to its normal resting state. This process is called *recovery*.

Recovery in nerve and isolated muscle tissue begins at the same point that excitation began. There is no evidence to indicate it does otherwise in cardiac muscle. Cardiac muscle fibers recover in a similar manner. As recovery progresses along the fiber, it forms a boundary at any one instant between recovered (resting) tissue and excited tissue (Fig. 23). This boundary is the *wave of recovery*. It has exactly the same characteristics as the wave of excitation. *A wave of recovery creates a force in the surrounding media directed toward the area of resting (recovered) tissue and away from excited tissue.*

THE WAVE FRONT

When a wave front is a flat surface, the force it creates is directly proportional to its area. Although the magnitude may be altered by

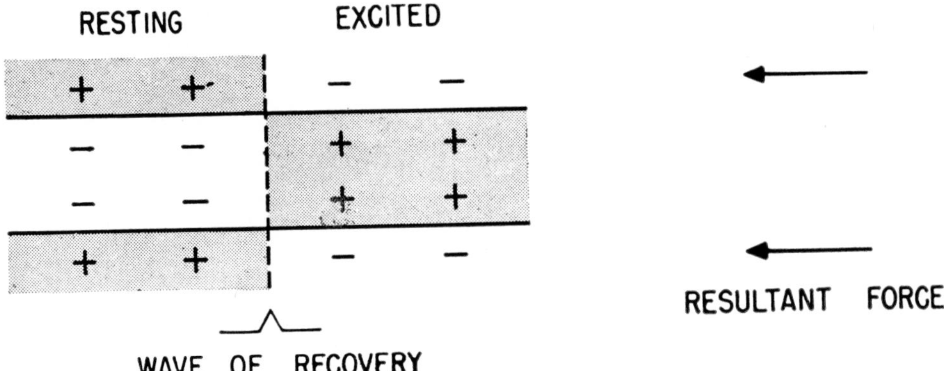

Figure 23.

changes in electrolytic and physical environment (the density of doublet charge), the relationship between wave area and magnitude persists. Thus the larger the flat surface area of the wave front, the larger the magnitude of the force (potential). The wave front may be regarded as having forces acting perpendicular to its surface at all points.

If the magnitude of the force created by the wave front is known in mv. and its duration of action in sec. is determined, its value can be expressed in mv. × sec. A force of 10 mv. across a wave front lasting 10 sec. is expressed as 100 mv. sec. Expression of potential differences acting through a period of time in this manner is frequently used in electrocardiography.

The wave front is not always flat. When it is not flat the force created in the surrounding media is no longer proportional to its surface area. Vector doublets will act perpendicular at all surface points. By vector addition, when forces are not acting parallel and in the same direction, the resultant of their action is not equivalent to the sum of their individual magnitude. *The effective force of a wave front is equivalent to the resultant of the doublet vectors acting perpendicular to its surface.*

Given a conical wave front one can calculate its resultant vector (Fig. 24). Since all the doublet vectors are acting perpendicular to the wave front their resultant will be perpendicular to the base (assuming even distribution of doublet charges). This exemplifies an important principle of wave fronts, *whenever a wave front bounds a single flat surface area its resultant will be perpendicular to the flat surface.* The magnitude of the resultant vector will be directly proportional to the area of the base. *Whenever a single flat surface area is bounded by a wave front, the magnitude of its resultant vector is directly proportional to the area of the flat surface.**

A wave front may have more than one flat surface area. A cone with ⅙ of its arc cut away

*This simple principle is verified by the theorem of Gauss. In part there are two essential equations. The electrical intensity at a point in field due to multiple distributions of electrical charge is found in the equation

$$\iint E \cos \Theta \, ds = \frac{4\pi}{k} Q.$$

The intensity (E) at a point on the surface distant to a field created by a uniformly charged spherical shell is

$$E = \frac{Q}{k\,r^2} \text{ dynes per stat coulomb.}$$

Q is the charge, k is the dielectric constant of the surrounding media and r is the distance between the surface point and the center of the spherical shell. It should be noted that effect of the spherical shell is as if the intensity originated from the center of the sphere. For further detail the reader is referred to: Gilbert, Norman E.: Electricity and Magnetism, Third Edition, New York, The Macmillan Company, 1950.

An equation by derivation from the work of Gauss was used by Wilson to calculate point potential at a distance from the source, $V = \phi S \frac{\cos \Theta}{r^2}$ where V was the point potential, ϕ the density of charge, S the flat surface area, Θ the angle between the axis of the flat disk and a line drawn to the potential point and r the distance between the point from the flat disk. Wilson, F. N., MacLeod, A. G., and Barker, P. S.: *The Distribution of the Currents of Action and Injury Displayed by Heart Muscle and other Excitable Tissues.* Univ. of Mich. Studies, Scientific Series, Ann Arbor, Univ. of Mich. Press, 1933, Vol. 18, p. 58.

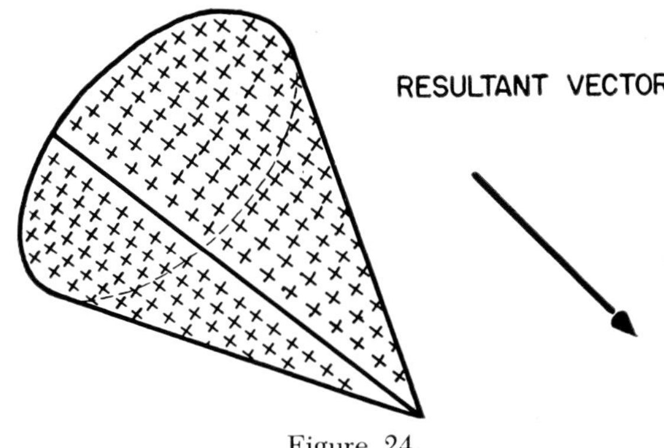

Figure 24.

has two flat surface areas (Fig. 25). The resultant of the wave front is equal to the resultant of two vectors, one representing the base of the cone and the other flat surface area created by the ⅙ conical arc.

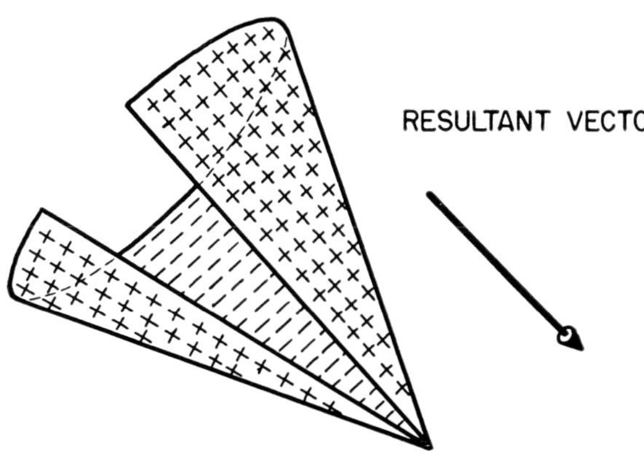

Figure 25.

SUMMARY OF NORMAL EXCITATION AND RECOVERY

The following simple rules may be formulated to summarize excitation and recovery of a normal muscle fiber:

1) Muscle fibers in the resting state create no effective external force.

2) Muscle fibers in the excited state create no effective external force.

3) The boundary between muscle areas in different electrical states (excited and resting) is a wave front and creates a force directed toward the area of muscle in the resting or recovered state.

4) The magnitude of the force created by a wave front is the resultant of the doublet vectors acting everywhere perpendicular to the wave front.

5) Under normal circumstances recovery begins at the same site as the onset of excitation. This creates a force opposite the force of excitation (rule 3).

FACTORS INFLUENCING CELLULAR RECOVERY

Recovery of the isolated muscle strip is very sensitive. Numerous factors may alter its usual process. Warming speeds up recovery. If one end of the muscle strip is warmed that end may recover first regardless of the original point of excitation. Cooling slows recovery. By cooling one end of the muscle strip one can delay recovery at that region. By decreasing the oxygen supply to a region of muscle it becomes hypoxic and recovery in that region will be delayed.

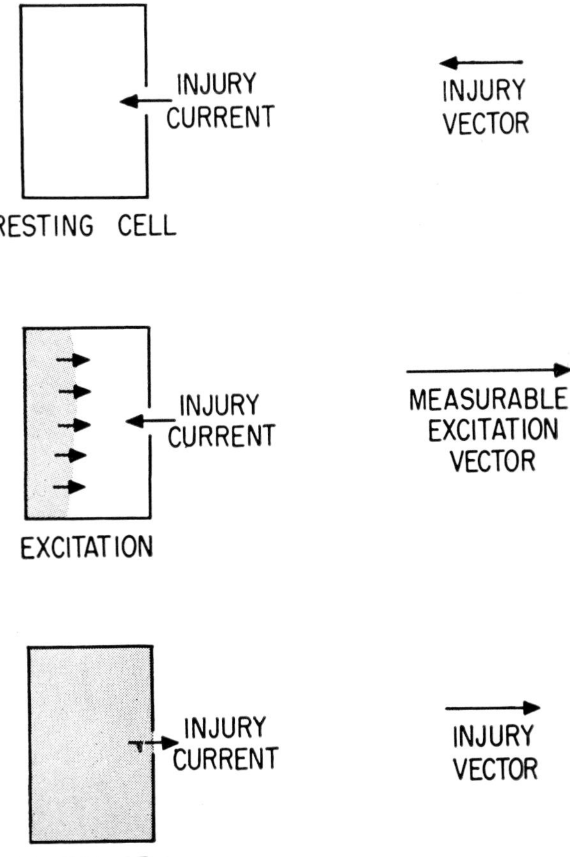

Figure 26.

Drugs can alter recovery by their chemical action on the cell membrane. Changes in the electrolyte content of the cellular media and in the fluids surrounding the media will alter the usual driving forces across the cell membrane and may profoundly affect both recovery and excitation.

EFFECTS OF CELL INJURY

Cell injury creates a constant force at the area of injury. Injury connotes the destruction of the cell membrane. This permits a constant diffusion of electrical current between the internal and external environment of the cell. In the resting state the external environment is relatively positive, therefore a constant flow from outside to inside exists through the area of injury (Fig. 26). Moreover the force across the membrane (resting membrane action potential) opposite the area of injury is unopposed. These forces create a vector towards the normal tissue area and away from the area of injury. The excited cell has a positive internal environment and creates a force toward the exterior. The membrane action potential is also reversed in the excited state. The resultant of these forces creates a vector toward the injured area during the excitation phase. Recording techniques are such that injury forces are measured only during the excited phase (between excitation and recovery). For this reason the injury vector is manifested only during excitation and the following rule may be formulated: *Injury creates a vector directed toward the area of injury.*

III

The Heart as a Source of Electrical Forces

ATRIAL EXCITATION

THE ATRIA are thin walled structures. The right atrium forms the right border of the heart and is anterior to the left atrium. The left atrium is the most posterior part of the heart and forms the right posterior chamber. Both are composed of muscle fibers giving them wall thickness. Like all resting cells a positive electrical field comprises the external environment. Of necessity both atrial surfaces (internal and external) are positive with respect to the cellular interior, during the resting state.

Excitation of the atria begins from a stimulus emitted by the sino-auricular node. This is a body of specialized conduction tissue situated at the orifices of the vena cava. It is a long narrow body. It is normally responsible for cardiac rate and is called the pacemaker. The node is subject to influences from the vagus nerve (chiefly, the right vagus) and the sympathetic nerve supply. The former slows the node's activity and can arrest its action completely, while the latter accelerates its activity.

The SA node is external to the atria, causing excitation to begin at the external surface. The wave of excitation spreads away from its point of origin. Its pathway over the external surface can be roughly described as a series of expanding concentric circles. Since the atria are thin walled structures, only a short time is required for excitation to reach the internal surface under normal circumstances. Nevertheless, the fact that time for transmission is required should not be overlooked. The time factor is of importance in pathological states. The early arrival of the wave of excitation at the inner surface prevents the wave of excitation from obtaining any large area (Fig. 27). This, in turn, prevents normal atrial excitation from creating a large force. Should transmission to the inner surface be delayed, the wave of excitation increases in size, creating a larger force. Those clinical conditions causing delay in transmission of the wave front are associated with increased electrical force, regardless of the presence or absence of atrial hypertrophy.

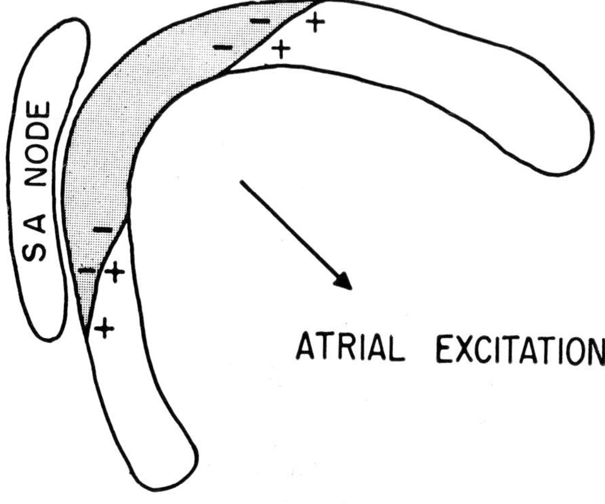

Figure 27.

The force created by atrial excitation begins with zero magnitude, increases to its maximum, and returns to zero. The resultant vector rotates its direction. The vector terminus of necessity describes a pathway in space, or a loop. This loop represents atrial excitation and is called the P loop. Atrial excitation involves the successive addition and subtraction of vector quantities. The spatial pathway then becomes an expression of magnitude of the forces of excitation. The pathway is small, as forces are being added and subtracted simultaneously. This is the result of the arrival of the excitation wave at the inner surface prior to completion of excitation of the external surface.

Since atrial excitation spreads away from the SA node, its force is directed away from the orifices of the vena cava. This is the old rule that the force of excitation is directed away from the excited area.

The time required for atrial excitation does not exceed .12 sec. The time interval depends upon the speed of radial transmission of excitation through the muscle fibers (3-5 mm. per .01 sec.) and the surface area of the atria. When the atrial volume is large the surface area to be excited is greater, thus prolonging atrial excitation.

VENTRICULAR EXCITATION

In order to appreciate the spatial direction of forces created by ventricular excitation, certain simple anatomic facts must be considered. 1) The left ventricle comprises the larger part of ventricular mass. It is shaped much like a cone. The base of this cone faces the right posterior chest. The apex of the cone is directed anteriorly and to the left. The cone rests on its side above the diaphragm. The wall of the cone is thickest at its base and becomes progressively thinner towards the apex. 2) The wall of the left ventricle is normally three or four times as thick as the wall of the right ventricle. 3) The margins of the free wall of the right ventricle are attached to the anterior surface of the left ventricular cone. The portion of the left ventricular wall bounded by this attachment represents the septum, or partition between the ventricular cavities. 4) The septum is anatomically and functionally part of the left ventricle. The segment of the cone comprising the septum is a 60° arc.* 5) The septum faces the anterior chest wall. The right ventricle, then, is anterior to the left ventricle (Fig. 28).

*Grant, R. P.: Architectonics of the heart. *Am. Heart J.* *46*:405, 1953.

At the base of the septum, next to the atria, is the AV node. This tissue is a bundle of specialized conduction tissue which transmits the electrical impulse from the atria to the ventricles. Normally there is a delay between atrial and ventricular excitation due to the time required for the transmission of the excitation impulse through this conduction pathway to its receptor end plates in the myocardium. The node has many ramifications of tissue fibers spreading over both surfaces of the septum and the entire endocardial cavities of both ventricles. This tissue transmits impulses very rapidly. It permits rapid excitation throughout the endocardial surfaces.

The order of excitation of the component portions of the ventricle is now relatively well understood. 1) The left endocardial surface of the septum is activated first. 2) About .005 sec. after the onset of excitation, the right endocardial septal surface is activated. 3) The remainder of both endocardial surfaces complete activation by .02 sec. after the onset of ventricular excitation. Thus, at .02 sec., excitation appears as two confluent cones of activity placed side by side. 4) Excitation spreads externally through the muscle thickness at a rate of 1/3 meter per sec. (3 mm. per .01 sec.). 5) The thin walled right ventricle completes activation first, normally between .020 and .040 sec. 6) The septum is activated from both right and left surfaces, completing activation in less than one half the time required for complete ventricular excitation. For an excitation cycle of .08 sec. duration, septal activation should be complete by .04 sec.* The septum creates a small force

*The concept of rapid endocardial excitation is not new. It was originally proposed by Einthoven (1908). Wilson made use of Einthoven's explanation and his comments relative to endocardial and septal activation are as follows: "Excitation of the subendocardial muscle begins at many different points almost simultaneously (6), so that many islands of active tissue, one for each junction between the Purkinje tissue and the ordinary muscle, are quickly formed. As these islands grow they coalesce to form larger islands, until both ventricular cavities are lined almost everywhere except at the orifices by a sheet of active muscle. At this stage of ventricular excitation there is a boundary between resting and active muscle in almost every part of the outside

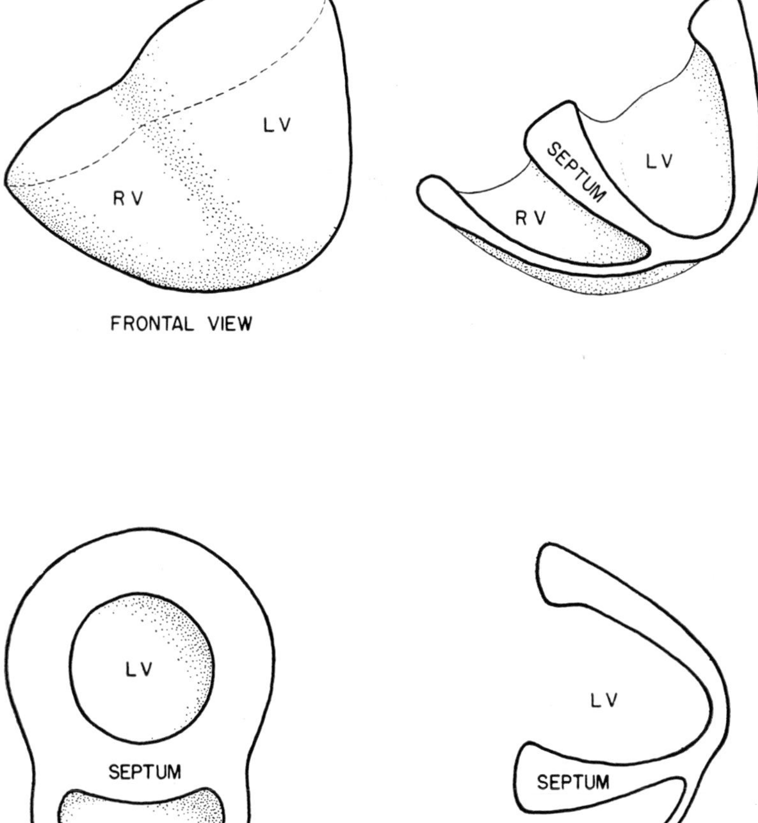

Figure 28.

of very short duration because it is activated nearly simultaneously from both sides. After completion of right ventricular and septal activation, the wave of excitation is only part of a cone of activity located in the left ventricle. It is a cone with an arc of 60° cut away from its wall. The 60° arc represents the septal region that has completed activation. 7) The cone, or wave front, becomes progressively shorter as new muscle areas complete activation. The cone is thinnest at the apex; thus, the wave front arrives first at the surface of the left ventricle, near the apex. It arrives at the surface at progressively later intervals from the apex to the base. The size of the wave front, then, is diminished from the apex to the base (Fig. 29).

The effective force of a wave of excitation is the resultant of the doublet vectors acting perpendicular to the wave front. With this principle in mind the resultant vector of the wave of excitation can be determined at any stage of the cycle. 1) The left septal surface begins activation creating a force directed away from the excited region. Considering the anatomic

walls; in the septum, which is activated from both sides, there are two such boundaries. The two groups of electrical forces associated with the two septal boundaries are opposite in direction and cancel one another more or less completely, so that the voltage across the septum is normally small." Wilson, F. N., Rosenbaum, F. F., and Johnston, F. D.: *Interpretation of the Ventricular Complex of the Electrocardiogram, Advances in Internal Medicine.* New York, Interscience Publishers, Inc., 1947, Vol. 2, pp. 1-63.

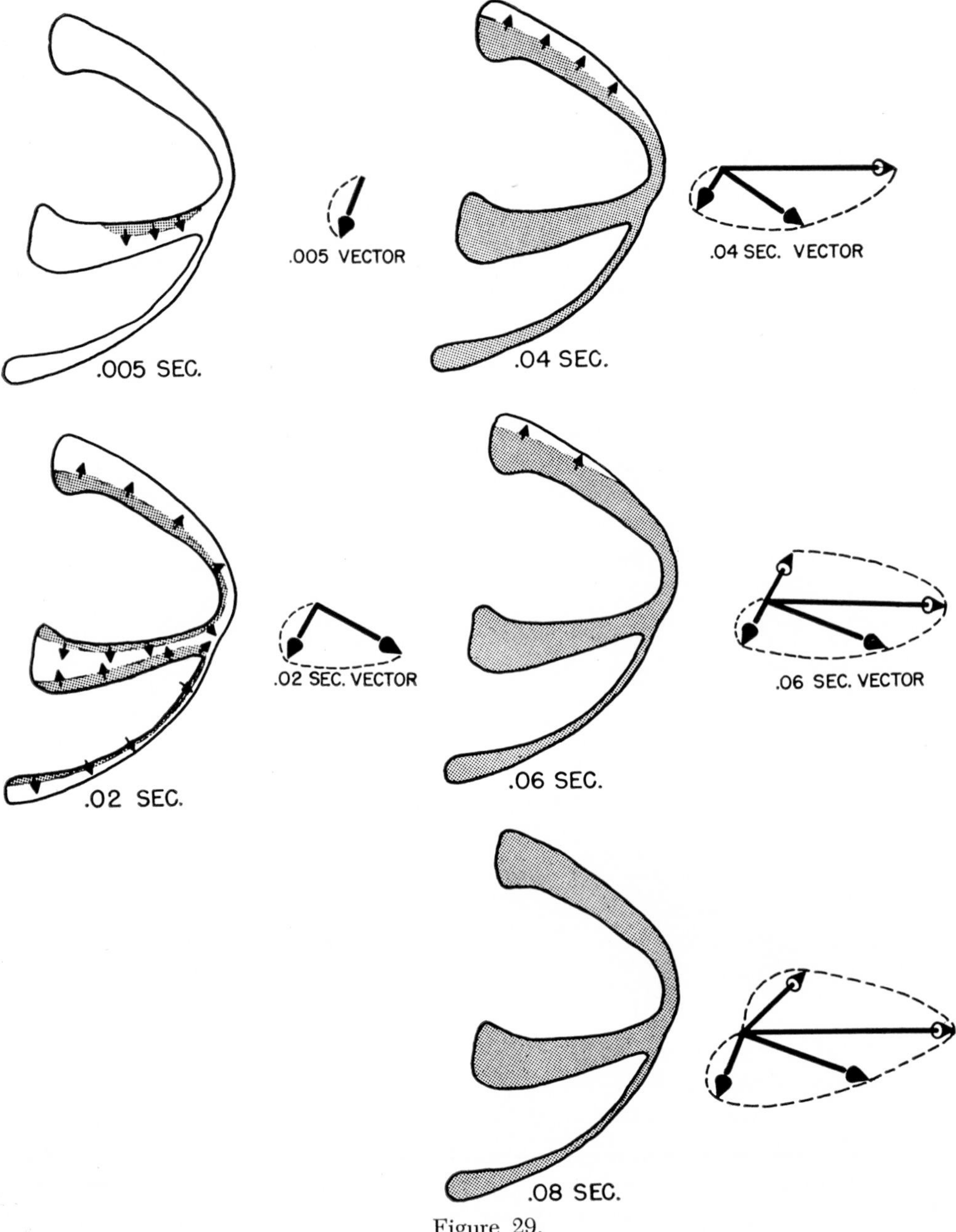

Figure 29.

location of the septum, this means the initial force is anterior and to the right. The duration of this unopposed force is .005 sec. At this time activation of the right septal surface begins and neutralizes the force from the left surface. 2) Endocardial spread continues in both cavities. When both cones are complete (.02 sec.) a flat surface area is bounded by the cones of excitation which is roughly equivalent to the base of the ventricles. The resultant vector is proportional to this area and perpendicular to the base of the heart. It should be parallel to the long axis of the ventricles, directed to the left and anteriorly. 3) Completion of activation of the right ventricular wall (.035 sec.) causes posterior rotation of the resultant vector. 4) As the wave front diminishes in size from apex to base, the resultant vector magnitude decreases.

The vector rotates backward as it becomes shorter. Its terminal location is roughly perpendicular to the long axis of the left ventricle.

The instantaneous vector at the completion of right ventricular activation is of special interest (usually about .035 sec. and usually the longest instantaneous spatial vector). It is the resultant of vectors representing two flat surface areas, the area of the base of the left ventricle and the flat surface area of the septum (Fig. 30). The term *long left ventricular vector* will be used to designate this vector. When the ventricle is a short cone the septal surface area is small and the long left ventricular vector is more nearly parallel to the long axis of the ventricles. As the ventricle elongates the septal area is increased causing the left ventricular vector to rotate more posteriorly away from the long axis of the ventricles.

The continuous rotation of the resultant vector describes a spatial pathway. The resultants are thought of as rotating upon a center of origin. For ventricular excitation this center is confined to a small area in the left ventricle. Its stationary characteristic is due to the shape of the wave front of excitation. For the most part, the wave front represents a cone, or a 300° arc of a cone. With all forces acting perpendicular to the wave front it is easy to understand why the lines of force all intersect a relatively small area. The validity of this concept will be further explored in the discussion of volume conductors.

The rotation of a central resultant on its point of origin is caused by the successive addition or subtraction of new vectors. The spatial pathway is a measure of the magnitude of newly added or subtracted forces. The pathway is the sides of a polygon. Because the events are rapid changes of small magnitude it becomes a loop. The magnitude of the force causing rotation from one central resultant position to another is the length of the spatial pathway. These principles are readily applied to ventricular excitation. The magnitude of the force acting to rotate the resultant vector from one position to another is equivalent to the distance between the two vector points, or that segment of the spatial pathway. The length of the pathway between the terminus of the .04 sec. vector and the .05 sec. vector represents the change of force acting between the .04 sec. interval and the .05 sec. interval. This force is proportional to the change in the area of the wave front between the .04 and.05 sec. intervals.

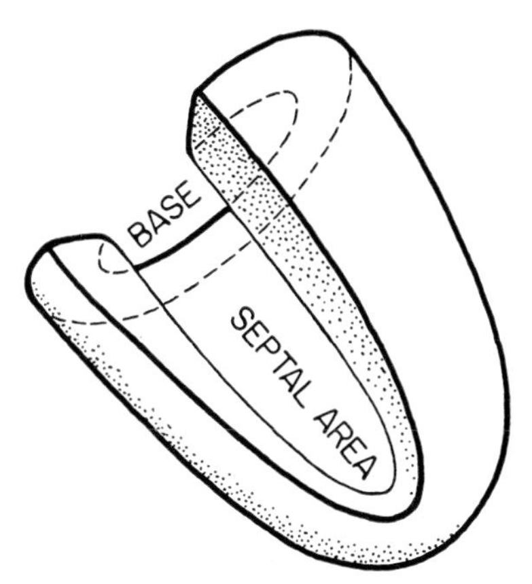

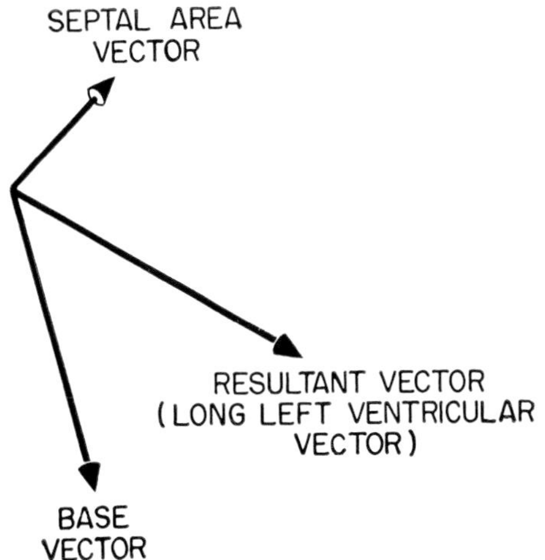

Figure 30.

The length of the spatial pathway between the long left ventricular vector and completion of ventricular excitation is an index of left ventricular surface area (and volume). This measurement can be determined by indirect means and will be called *the index of maximum potential for the left ventricle.* It has a direct relationship to the long left ventricular vector.

The apical segments of the wave of excitation have a shorter duration of action than the basilar region. The duration of action for the conical wave front segment lost from .04 to .05 sec., averages .04 to .05* To express the potential in terms of duration of action represented by this conical segment in time units one can multiply the length of the spatial pathway from .04 to .05 sec. by .045 sec. The product is expressed in mv. × sec./100.

An expression of the *potential seconds* for the conical segment represented by the time interval .05 to .06 can be obtained in a similar manner as above. After determining the mv. × sec./100 for each conical segment they may be added. The sum is an index of the potential × sec./100 created by left ventricular excitation and may be called the *potential seconds for the left ventricle per cardiac cycle.* It is an expression of the surface area of the ventricle, the thickness of the muscle wall and the density of electrical charges across the wave front.†

There is a marked increase in wall thickness at the base of the ventricles. This causes slow changes in the size of the wave front, and terminal slowing of the spatial pathway described by the rotating instantaneous spatial resultant vector. This area creates further complications because it is not always well supplied with specialized conduction tissue. As a result activation may be somewhat delayed and create terminal variations in the direction of excitation forces.

VENTRICULAR RECOVERY

The isolated muscle strip begins recovery at the same site as the onset of excitation. The ventricle behaves in an exactly similar fashion. The thin walled right ventricle begins recovery at its apex, shortly or immediately after completion of ventricular excitation. The apex region of the left ventricle then begins recovery, at its endocardial region.* Recovery proceeds from apex to base. The usual time required for recovery is between .26 and .36 sec. depending upon cardiac rate.

Since the force across a wave front is always directed towards the resting (recovered) tissue, the spatial forces of ventricular recovery can be analyzed. Initial apical recovery of the right ventricular wall creates a force anteriorly and leftward. This force is small because the area of the wave front is small. Recovery of the left ventricle from apex to base creates a force directed away from the base, to the left and anterior. The magnitude of the force depends upon both the shape and size of the wave front of recovery. Normally it is smaller than the forces of excitation. The forces of recovery are roughly parallel to the long axis of the heart.

The important point about ventricular recovery is its onset at the apex. The base apex relationship to ventricular recovery was clearly demonstrated by Mines† in 1913, by means of a base apex lead. He observed that warming of the base of the heart created a negative T wave. A negative T wave was made positive by apical warming. Cooling of the apex produced a negative T wave. He correctly attributed these findings to change in speed of recovery, increased with warming and slowed with cooling. Later, Wilson and Herrmann (1921)§ demonstrated

*Actually. 01 or .015 sec. should be subtracted from the time interval for the time required for endocardial activation but for practical purposes this small period of delay may be ignored.

†Actual calculation of total potential would require conversion by geometric factors related to the length of the ventricle and the area of the base as used in conic calculations.

*The initial recovery of the endocardium is responsible for the negative force of recovery following the upright excitation wave as recorded directly from the surface of the heart muscle. Sir Thomas Lewis demonstrated this pattern and called it an electrogram. Recent interest in this observation has been revived since its frequent demonstration during cardial surgery. The area of muscle beneath the electrode is to be regarded as an isolated muscle strip. Lewis, Thomas: *The Mechanism and Graphic Registration of the Heart Beat.* New York, Paul B. Hoeber, Inc. 1920.

†Mines, G. R.: On functional analysis by the action of electrolytes. *J. Physiol., 46:*188, 1913.

§These classic experiments were done in experimental bundle branch block. The end of the refractory period was correlated with the decline in excitation. In right bundle branch block the left ventricle passed out of the refractory state .02 to .04 sec. before the right ventricle. The deeper

that recovery followed the same general order as excitation.

A popular theoretical explanation for the direction of the forces of ventricular recovery is delay in recovery of the endocardial regions. This concept is without experimental support. It is contrary to known experimental observations. As long as apical recovery occurs first the resultant vector will be directed away from the base regardless of whether recovery begins at the endocardial or epicardial surface (Fig. 31).

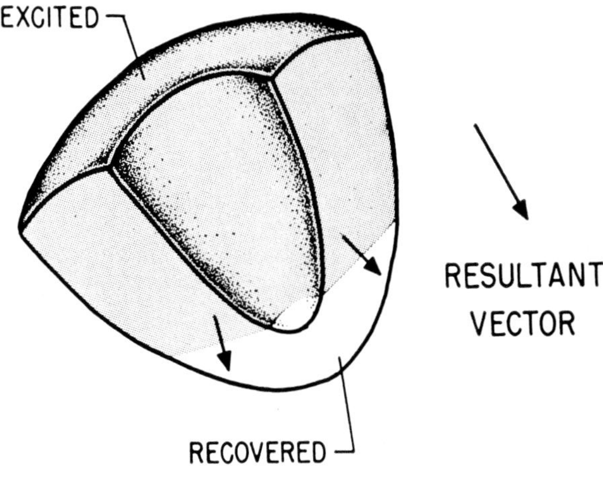

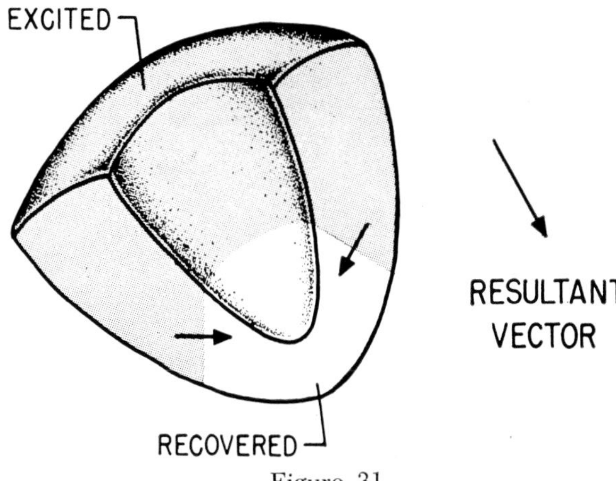

Figure 31.

The wave front of recovery closely resembles a complete conical segment (360°). A change in the inclination of the walls of the cone greatly alters the resultant vector magnitude. A cylin-

layers of the left apex passed out of the refractory state before the surface layers. The right ventricle recovered before the left ventricle in the presence of right bundle branch block. On the basis of these observations the authors stated, "We have shown that the order of recovery of the various regions of the ventricular mass is the same as the order of excitation." Wilson, F. N., and Herrmann, G. R.: An experimental study of incomplete bundle branch block and of the refractory period of the heart of the dog. *Heart*, *8*:229, 1921.

Dr. Herrmann has been kind enough to review the concept of the base apex relation in production of the T wave and is in agreement with the concept set forth.

The concept of the ventricular gradient was ushered into electrocardiography as a pure theoretical paper presented by Wilson in 1931. It is of interest to note that he defined the "ventricular gradient" as the mean electrical axis of Q-R-S-T, which pointed away from the ventricular region with the longest average duration of excitation and towards the region of least average duration. He pointed out that the normal ventricular gradient pointed in a base apex direction because tthe average length of systole was greater at the base than at the apex. Wilson, F. N., MacLeod, A. G., and Barker, P. S.: The T deflection of the electrocardiogram, *Tr. A. Am. Physicians*, *46*:29, 1931.

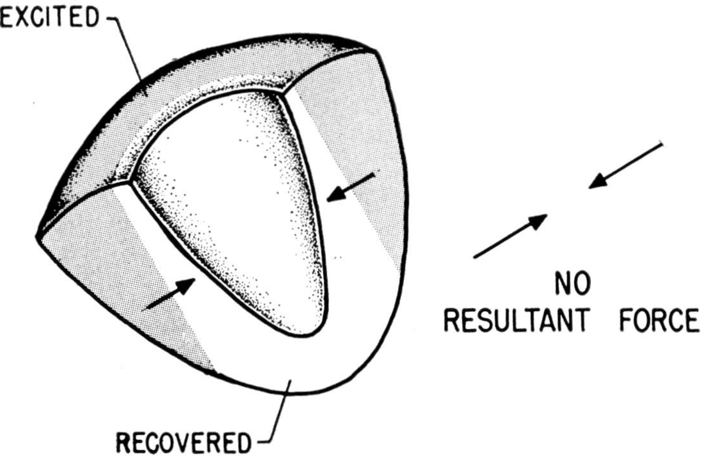

Figure 32.

drical wave front creates forces opposed to each other. The resultant approaches zero magnitude. This is one explanation for demonstration of excitation forces and absence of demonstrable recovery forces (Fig. 32). The creation of an everted conical wave front reverses the customary direction of recovery forces. The resultant vector is directed toward the base rather than toward the apex (Fig. 33).

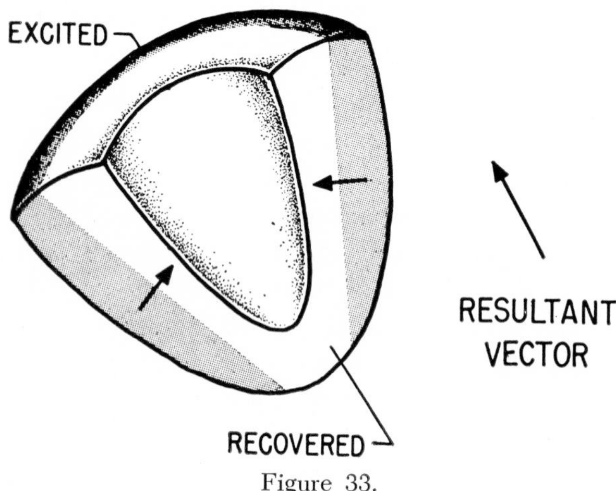

Figure 33.

The normal course of recovery creates a continuously changing vector describing a loop. The loop is enclosed within the QRS loop and is smaller in magnitude. Commonly it is somewhat anterior to the point of origin. It is called the T loop. Its spatial pathway is a function of the magnitude of the component forces. Since there is a continuous loss of forces at the same time of addition of new forces the spatial pathway is small in comparison to the QRS pathway. The T loop appears somewhat anterior to the QRS loop because the latter has a long posterior course caused by early completion of septal activation.

AFTER POTENTIAL

A small additional wave of electrical activity may follow ventricular recovery. This event is called the U event. Its cause is not completely understood. It will also describe a spatial pathway and its forces are roughly parallel to the forces of ventricular recovery.

IV

Fundamentals of Conductors

CHARACTERISTICS OF CONDUCTORS

A CONDUCTOR is a medium for the transmission of electricity. When a complete circuit exists, current flows through a conductor. The media serving as a conductor offers resistance to the transmission of electrical force. When the resistance is great the forces are poorly transmitted. Such a media is a poor conductor. A media offering little resistance to transmission of forces is a good conductor. In a general sense all substances are conductors. However, some are such poor conductors that a very large force must be present to transmit electrical forces any great distance from the source. Such substances are called insulators. Wood, air and rubber are examples of poor conductors. Copper and zinc are examples of good conductors.

Conductors may be either solid, gas or liquid. A volume of liquid used as a conductor is called a volume conductor. Water is a good conductor when it contains electrolytes, the greater the concentration of electrolytes the better its conductivity.

When a conductor offers a uniform amount of resistance to electrical forces throughout, it is called a *homogeneous conductor*. In such a conductor, if one knows the amount of resistance offered by 1 centimeter of distance from the source, one can calculate the total resistance offered at any distance from the source. A conductor which does not offer a uniform resistance throughout is called a *heterogeneous conductor*. Due to the variation in resistance at different areas, the total resistance cannot be determined in the same manner as for a homogeneous conductor.

ELECTRICAL FIELD WITHIN A VOLUME CONDUCTOR

An electrical field is created around a charged particle within a volume conductor. Potential diminishes as the distance from the particle (source) is increased. In volume conductors the potential diminishes in proportion to the square of the radius distance (r^2). This is due to the spherical dissipation of the force. In a flat disk conductor, potential diminishes simply in relation to the radius distance (r).

The presence of two fields of unequal potential (positive and negative) creates a resultant force. The direction of this force is a straight line drawn from the point of lowest potential (negative pole) to the point of greatest potential (positive pole). The force may be represented as a vector directed toward the positive pole and away from the negative pole. This vector represents the axis of the electrical field. It is the dipole vector (or doublet vector). The magnitude of the dipole vector depends upon the difference in potential between the two poles and is called the dipole moment (electrical moment).

In electrocardiography we are concerned with a negative field on one side of a wave front and a positive field on the opposite side. The magnitude of the dipole moment (electrical moment) depends upon the density of charges (doublet vectors) and the flat surface area of the wave front. It is then an expression of the effective force created by the wave front.

INFINITE VOLUME CONDUCTORS

At any point within an infinite volume conductor the potential depends upon: 1) the magnitude of the dipole vector or electrical moment, M, 2) the distance of the point from the center of origin, r, and 3) the angle between the dipole vector and the coordinate drawn from the potential point and the center of origin (Fig. 34). This may be expressed as a simple equation:

$$\text{Potential} = M \frac{\cos \Theta}{r^2} .$$

If one measures the potential and knows angle Θ and the radius distance, the dipole moment, M, can be determined.

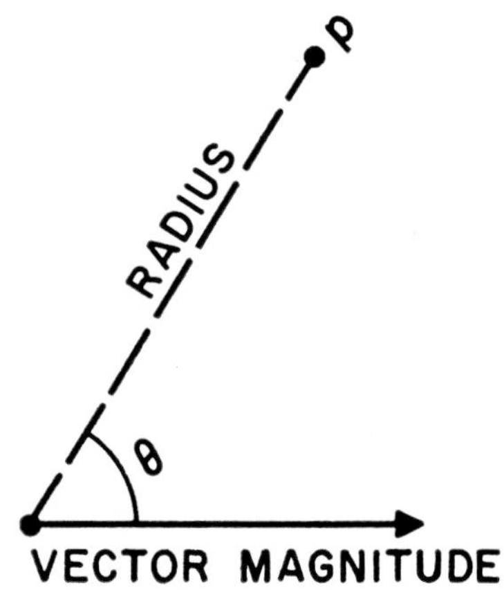

Figure 34.

FINITE VOLUME CONDUCTORS

The potential is always greater at the surface of a limited volume conductor than it would be at the same distance from the source in an infinite volume conductor. This is due to the insulating effect of the surface. These effects are not so noticeable near the center of a tank. For a spherical type tank it has been determined that the potential is approximately three times as great at the surface as would be expected for that distance. This is particularly important in electrocardiography as measurements are made from the surface. The potential at the surface of a spherical finite volume conductor is expressed:*

$$\text{Potential} = 3 \times M \frac{\cos \Theta}{r^2} .$$

The shape of the boundary also influences the potential measurement. A rectangular tank will distort the apparent direction of the dipole vector. Variations in resistance within the volume conductor will further distort the direction of the lines of force and alter potential measurements.

*Wilson, F. N., MacLeod, A. G., and Barker, P. S.: *The Distribution of the Currents of Action and Injury Displayed by Heart Muscle and other Excitable Tissues.* Univ. of Mich. Studies, Scientific Series, Ann Arbor, Univ. of Mich. Press, 1933, Vol. 18, p. 58.

". . . at any point upon the surface of the sphere the magnitude of V is three times as great as it would be at the same point in an infinite medium."

THE BODY AS A VOLUME CONDUCTOR

For practical application it has been found convenient to consider the body as a homogeneous volume conductor. The body, consisting primarily of water and electrolytes, is a good volume conductor. It is true that resistance is not uniform throughout the body. Even the resistance offered by the skin varies at different points. The change in the character of the tissues alters the resistance factor. The air in the lungs is considered to act as an insulator. On the other hand, the lungs are highly vascular, and vascular beds are extremely good conductors. There are sources other than the heart creating electrical fields. In actuality then, the body is a heterogeneous volume conductor of variable resistances with multiple sources of electrical fields. In application, considering the body as a homogeneous volume conductor has been surprisingly satisfactory. Since this is a simple practical approach it shall be so considered here.

The wave front sets up an electrical field in the body. The isopotential plane defined on the body is perpendicular to the resultant vector of the wave front. The potential at any one point on the body is expressed by the equation:

$$\text{Potential} = 3 \times M \frac{\cos \Theta}{r^2} .$$

By locating the isopotential plane one can estimate the direction of the resultant vector. It is perpendicular to this plane. Errors due to variation in resistance and shape of the finite boundary are assumed.

LOCATION OF THE ZERO CENTER

A perplexing problem in electrocardiography concerns the location of the zero center within the volume conductor (body). Much of the earlier work was based on the principle of the centric placed zero center. Ample evidence exists proving the zero center is actually eccentric in position. Moreover, its eccentric location is a large factor in measuring potential at the surface of the body. There is no system of electrocardiography currently employed that avoids this error. This point will be discussed further in considering the lead systems.

Although considerable variation exists the zero center for ventricular excitation is usually three to four centimeters left of the mid sternal line, about the lower level of the fourth intercostal space, and one third the distance of the anterior posterior diameter of the chest from the sternum (Fig. 35). The anterior location of the center should be no surprise to those who have examined a sagittal X-ray of the chest. The mediastinum is clearly seen to occupy the anterior one third compartment, the remainder being composed of muscle and bone.

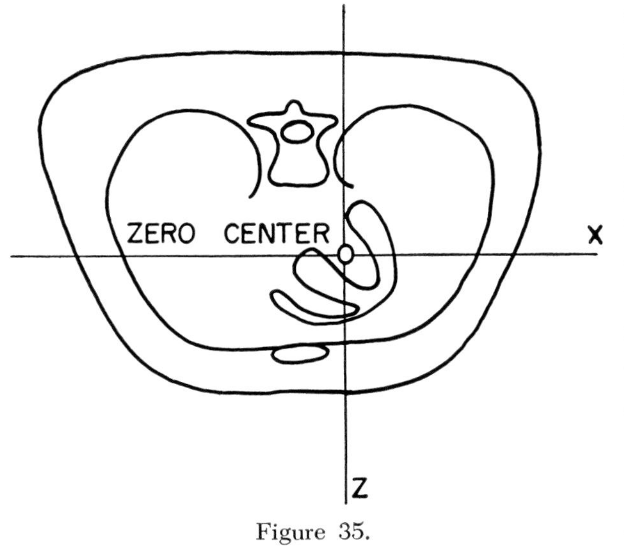

Figure 35.

REMOTE ELECTRODE AND PARTIAL LEAD EFFECT

Another complication in measuring potential from the surface of the body arises from the so-called "partial lead" effect. The implication is that potential values at points close to the heart are largely influenced by the nearest segment of muscle, rather than by the entire muscle mass. A point sufficiently distant from the heart not to be influenced by proximal muscle segments is called "remote." Both the diameter of the heart and distance from the heart determine whether a site is remote or not. Consider two doublet vectors of the heart in relation to a point *P* (Fig. 36). When the diameter of the heart is small the difference in radius distance from *P* to the doublet vectors is proportionally not so great.

The effect of distance is enhanced by resistance. A conductor of low resistance would require greater distances from the source to be a remote site. Experiments on the isolated perfused mammalian heart immersed in a volume conductor have been carried out.* Such experiments indicate that beyond distances of two to three times the diameter of the heart the site can be considered as remote. These studies verify the concept of a center of origin for the forces created by the heart when recorded at distances great enough to be considered remote.

*Hartmann, I., Veyrat, R., Wyss, Oscar A. M., and Duchosal, P. W.: Vectorcardiography as studied on the isolated mammalian heart suspended in a volume conductor. *Cardiologia, 27*:129, 1955.

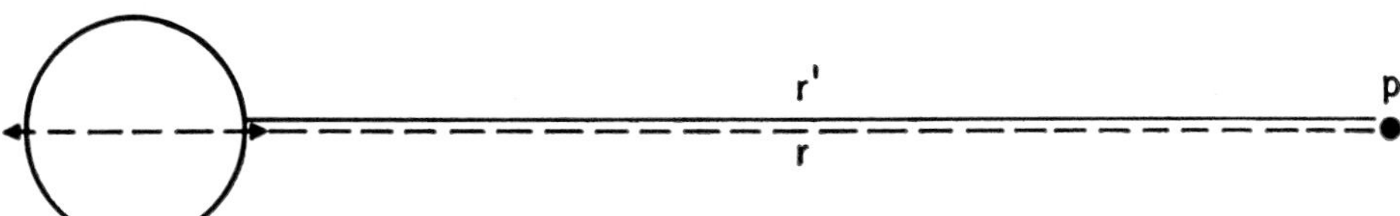

Figure 36.

V

Fundamentals of Electrocardiographic Instruments

THE PREVIOUS DISCUSSIONS have indicated that electrical fields are created by the heart, as a source, in a volume conductor, the body. At all points on the body surface potential exists due to the cardiac electrical cycle. These areas of potential have values which have a direct relationship to the heart and the character of the volume conductors. When the potential values on the body surface are known, the electrical activity of the heart can be ascertained. The next step is, logically, an instrument capable of measuring these potential values. To this end, three major types of recording devices are employed, the string gauge galvanometer with photographic recording system, the galvanometer with direct writing, recording system, and the cathode ray oscilloscope.

STRING GAUGE GALVANOMETER

The string gauge galvanometer consists of a conductor suspended between the two poles of an electromagnet. The conductor is a quartz glass fiber coated with platinum. The electromagnet sets up an electrical field. When an electric current passes through the conductor, the string is moved up or down in accordance with the principles of Fleming's law. One can illustrate this principle with the right hand (Fig. 37). The third, fourth and fifth fingers are pointed in the direction of force between the two poles of the electromagnet. The index finger is pointed in the direction of current flow through the suspended conductor. The extended thumb indicates the upward displacement of the conductor. If the direction of current is reversed through the conductor, it is deflected downward.

If electrical flow enters one terminal of the conductor a positive, or upward, displacement occurs. This terminal of the conductor is designated as the positive terminal, or the positive

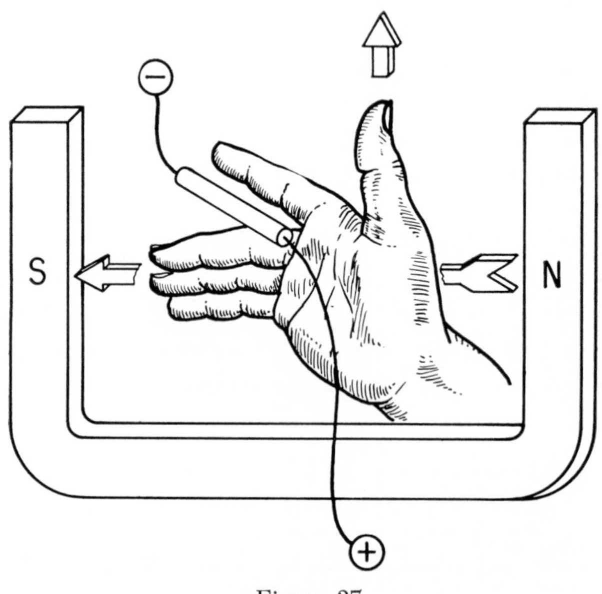

Figure 37.

electrode. Current entering the other terminal of the conductor causes a downward displacement. This terminal is designated as the negative electrode. The amount of displacement of the filament is dependent upon the difference in potential at each end of the conductor. The principle of the galvanometer may be summarized as follows: *A positive force entering the positive terminal (electrode) records a positive displacement.*

The string gauge galvanometer is considerably more reliable than the direct writing instruments, and for precise work it is much superior. It has been replaced largely because of the difficulties encountered in maintaining its day to day operation. The string, properly adjusted, offers little impedance to displacement and, as a consequence, there is little lag. To record the early events of septal activation, lag should be less than .001 sec.

The string gauge galvanometer records deflections of the string upon a moving film strip. The film strip may be marked at time intervals by spoke wheels or prisms. Usually the film is moved at 25 mm. per sec. Faster speeds are frequently an adjunct, and 50 mm. per sec. is commonly utilized. A vertical marker is indicated on the film at each .04 sec. interval. At each .20 sec. interval a heavier marker is indicated. It is always the fifth vertical marker. At a speed of 25 mm. per sec., the markers are one mm. apart. At 50 mm. per sec., they are two mm. apart. In either case they represent .04 sec.

The deflection of the string is the means of measuring the magnitude of the force for any lead. For standardization, one mm. is applied to the conductor. At full standardization this produces one cm. displacement of the string.

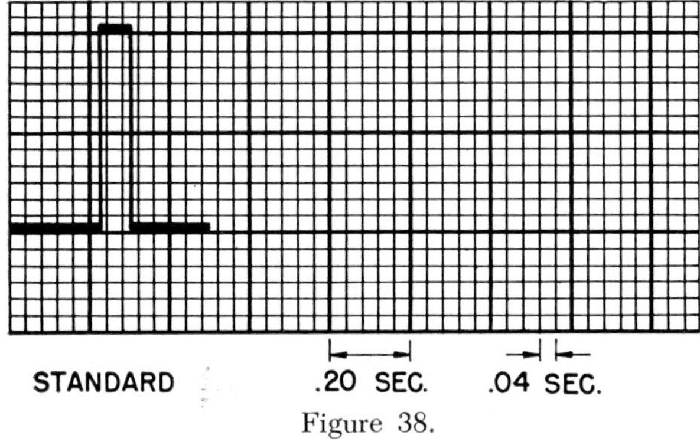

Figure 38.

This is an index of the sensitivity of the galvanometer (Fig. 38). When the sensitivity is known, any displacement of the string can be measured in millivolts. If it is not known, such measurements cannot be made. Frequently portions of records are recorded at "half standards," one millivolt producing ½ cm. deflection.

THE DIRECT WRITING INSTRUMENT

The direct writing instruments utilize the principle of the string gauge galvanometer, but the conductor and writing arm are heavy and the contact of the writing arm itself creates impedance to displacement. In a number of clinical conditions this is a serious handicap as it may obscure significant *Q* waves or small *R* waves. The peak of response to a force may be delayed from .01 to .015 sec. From the earlier discussion of rapid ventricular excitation it is clear that such measurements leave much to be desired. The direct writing instrument utilizes paper that is already graphed; the vertical lines are one mm. apart. At a speed of 25 mm. per sec. each square equals .04 sec. The writing arm should not be permitted to record in the bottom or top ½ cm. of the graph for most instruments.* The swing of the writing arm is damped at the limits of its excursion. The damping distorts (diminishes) the actual magnitude of the deflection.

CATHODE RAY OSCILLOSCOPE

The third type of recording instrument, and in my opinion the best, is the cathode ray oscilloscope (Fig. 39). It is a good instrument and has an excellent frequency response and no appreciable lag. The cathode ray tube emits an electron beam to the screen of the tube. On one side of the beam is a positive plate and opposite it is a negative plate. Any change in potential on the plates causes a movement of the beam. A second pair of plates is placed perpendicular to the first pair. Either pair may be used to record the potential difference between two points. The instrument may be standardized (per mv.) in a manner similar to the string gauge galvanometer. In addition to re-

*The Cambridge Simpliscribe is an exception.

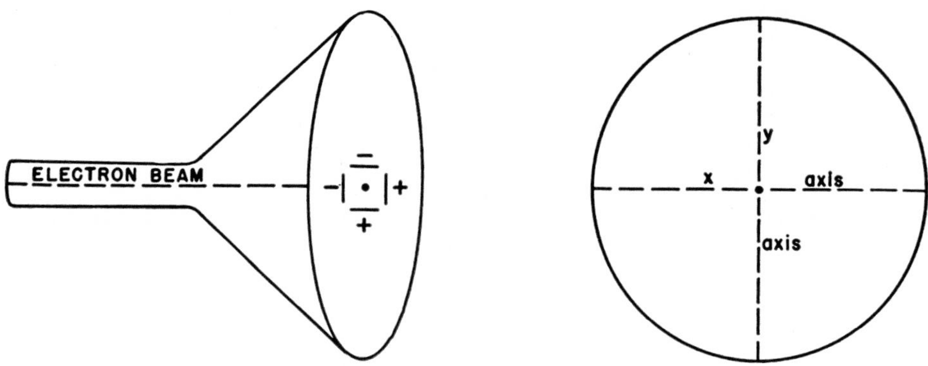

Figure 39.

cording an ordinary ECG, the presence of two perpendicular pairs of plates permits the use of this instrument for recording vector cardiograms which will be discussed more fully at another point in the text.

As a minimum standard, any of the instruments should have the following specifications:

1) Frequency response: With an input voltage of 15 cycles per sec., an output response of 90% of the input should be obtained. With an input voltage of 40 cycles per sec., the output response should be 80% of the input.

2) Linear response: When one mv. is applied, the peak response should be reached at .01 sec. It should be maintained at this peak, plus or minus 10% for 0.2 sec.

VI

Fundamentals of Electrocardiographic Leads

By utilizing the instruments for measuring potential at different points one can obtain an indirect measurement of the electrical events of the heart. The points selected for potential measurement have been standardized and constitute the lead systems used in electrocardiography. Any lead may be analyzed if the basic principles of potential measurement are properly applied.

EINTHOVEN'S LEADS

Einthoven originally measured potential at three points; left arm, right arm, and left leg. The difference in potential between these three points constitute Leads I, II, and III. It was assumed that all three potential points were equidistant from the zero center and equally distant from each other. Such leads are true bipolar or balanced leads. The extremities are considered as extensions of the lead wires. Thus, the potential is measured at the surface of the trunk (the volume conductor). The potential (V) points are then designated as from each shoulder (Vl and Vr), and foot (Vf).

Given a spatial vector with a point of origin equally distant from the potential points, Vl minus Vr will measure only the potential difference proportional to the X component of the spatial vector. The Y component of the spatial vector has the same effect upon positions Vl and Vr. If Vr is a negative electrode and Vl a positive electrode, they cancel each other, recording no potential difference due to the vertical component, –5 – (–5) = 0. The same principle applies to the sagittal component. Such a lead measures only the X component of the spatial vector and it is an X coordinate (Fig. 40). The magnitude of the vector measured by the lead is equal to: X vector component magnitude times $\frac{3L}{r^3}$, where L is the length of the lead (distance between Vl and Vr) and *r*

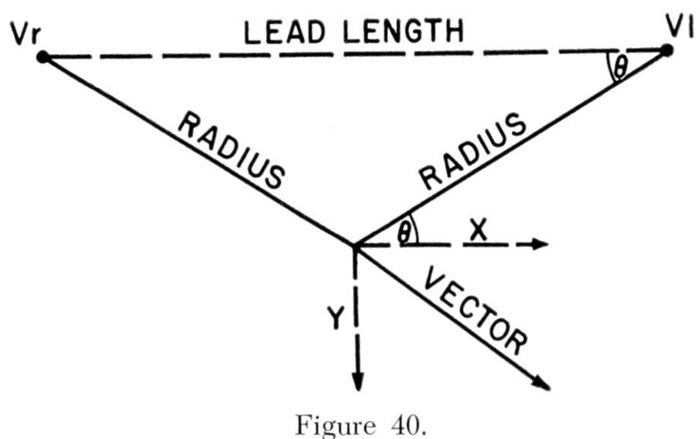

Figure 40.

is the radius distance between the point of origin and Vr or Vl.*

$$\text{Potential} = \text{Vector Magnitude} \times 3\,\frac{\cos\Theta}{r^2}$$

$$\cos\Theta = \frac{\frac{1}{2}L}{r}$$

or the potential at a given point, Vl, equals

$$3\left(\frac{\frac{1}{2}L}{r} \times \frac{1}{r^2}\right) = 3\left(\frac{\frac{1}{2}L}{r^3}\right)$$

$$\text{the potential at Vr} = -3\left(\frac{\frac{1}{2}L}{r^3}\right)$$

$$\text{Vl} - \text{Vr} = 3\left(\frac{\frac{1}{2}L}{r^3}\right) - \left(-3 \times \frac{\frac{1}{2}L}{r^3}\right) \text{ or } 3L/r.^3$$

The derivation of these simple equations demonstrates that a true bipolar lead measures potential magnitude in accordance with the radius distance and lead length. When these measure-

*This is from the formula of point potential at the surface of a spherical volume conductor:

ments are known it is possible to determine the relative magnitude of the vector component as it exists at the point of origin, within the volume conductor.*

EINTHOVEN'S TRIANGLE

Considering all three potential points (Vr, Vl, Vf) as equally distant from the zero center and of equal distance from each other, they describe an equilateral triangle (Fig. 41). This is called Einthoven's triangle. Lead I, with a positive electrode at Vl and a negative electrode at

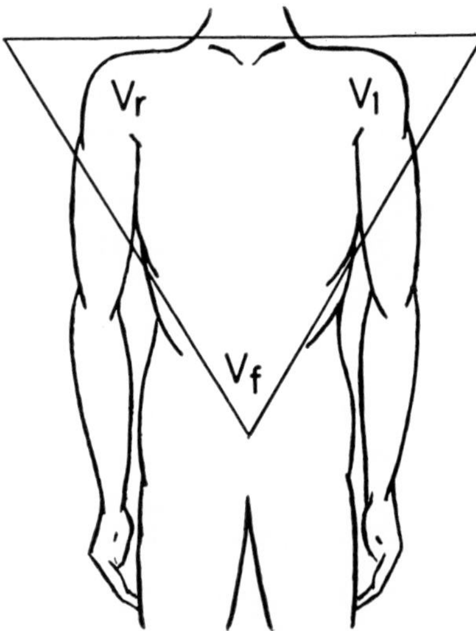

Figure 41.

Vr, measures potential Vl-Vr. Lead II, with a positive electrode at Vf and a negative electrode at Vr, measures potential Vf-Vr. Lead III, with a positive electrode at Vf and a negative electrode at Vl, measures potential Vf-Vl. The Einthoven triangle describes a circumstance wherein $3L/r^3$ is the same for each lead. Each lead is a coordinate.

EINTHOVEN'S LAW

A relationship exists between the three leads which is expressed as Einthoven's law: Lead I + Lead III = Lead II. This may be stated: (Vl-Vr + (Vf-Vl = (Vf-Vr). Einthoven's Law may be proved by assigning arbitrary values for the potential at each of the three points. If the potential at Vl is +5, Vr −10, and Vf +15, the law states:

Lead I = Vl-Vr = + 5 − (−10) = 5+10 or +15
Lead III = Vf-Vl = +15 − (+5) = 15 − 5 or +10

Lead II = Vf-Vr = + 15 − (−10) = + 15+10 or +25

THE BIPOLAR TRIAXIAL REFERENCE SYSTEM

The leads comprising Einthoven's triangle may be rearranged geometrically to form a Triaxial Reference System. Each of the three leads are bipolar with a positive and negative electrode located at different points on the volume conductor. At a point between the two electrodes there is an isopotential point. This point is located by constructing a perpendicular from the lead axis to the center of zero potential. The perpendicular intersects the isopotential point, or the point of origin for the lead. If the three points of origin for Leads I, II, and III are superimposed, a Triaxial Reference System is formed (Fig. 42). Since the original triangle

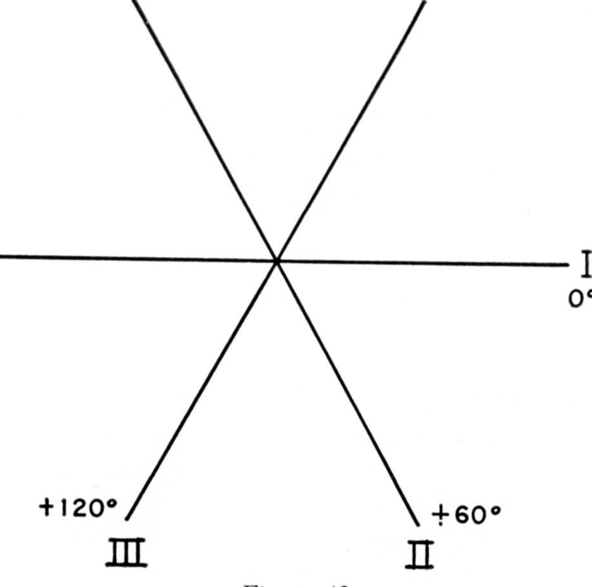

Figure 42.

was equilateral with angles of 60°, the angles formed about the center of origin of the Triaxial Reference System will also be 60°. The point of origin of the Triaxial Reference System is considered as superimposed on the center of zero

*This is a relative value as resistance is not known.

potential within the chest. This is valid as each lead has the same relative sensitivity, i.e., each lead records $3L/r^3$ times the actual force acting at the zero center.

For purposes of uniform orientation, Lead I has been designated as an axis of zero degrees. All points below Lead I are spoken of as positive degrees away from Lead I. All points above Lead I are spoken of as negative degrees away from Lead I. Thus, the positive pole of Lead II is +60° and the positive pole of Lead III is +120°.

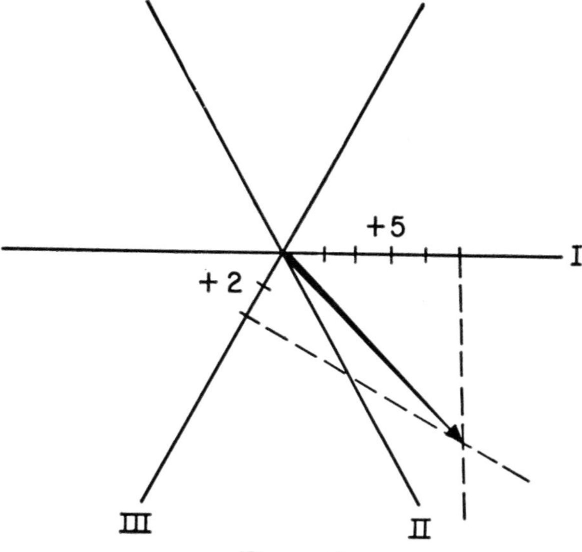

Figure 43.

LAW OF PARALLELOGRAMS

The direction and magnitude of a vector originating from the zero center can be calculated from its projection on any two leads. This is done by utilizing the Law of Parallelograms. If the vector registers a positive value of +5 in Lead I, and a value of +2 in Lead III, this is done as follows: 1) Mark off five units from the point of origin towards the positive pole of Lead I. 2) Construct a perpendicular from Lead I at this point. 3) Mark off two units from the point of origin, towards the positive pole of Lead III. 4) Construct a perpendicular from Lead III at this point. The two perpendicular lines will intersect one another. 5) A line is drawn from the point of origin of the reference system to the point of intersection by the two perpendicular lines. This line represents the direction and magnitude of the unknown vector. The vector is the diagonal of a parallelogram (Fig. 43).

The above process may be reversed. If the direction and magnitude of a vector is known, one can calculate its projection on any one of the three lead axes. The direction of the vector is defined in degrees away from the axis of Lead I.

A vector with a magnitude of +6, and an axis of +60° will be parallel to Lead II. It may be represented by marking off 6 units upon Lead II. A line constructed from this point on Lead II to a point perpendicular to Lead I, will designate 3 positive units on Lead I. A second line drawn from the terminal point of the force on Lead II to a point perpendicular to Lead III will designate 3 positive units on Lead III. The value of the vector projected on both Lead I and Lead III will be +3 units, conforming to Einthoven's Law, I + III = II, or +3 +3 = +6. This also illustrates an important characteristic of a vector, *the lead most nearly parallel to a vector will record the largest deflection* (Fig. 44).

A vector with an axis of +90° and a magnitude of 6 units will record 5 units in Lead II

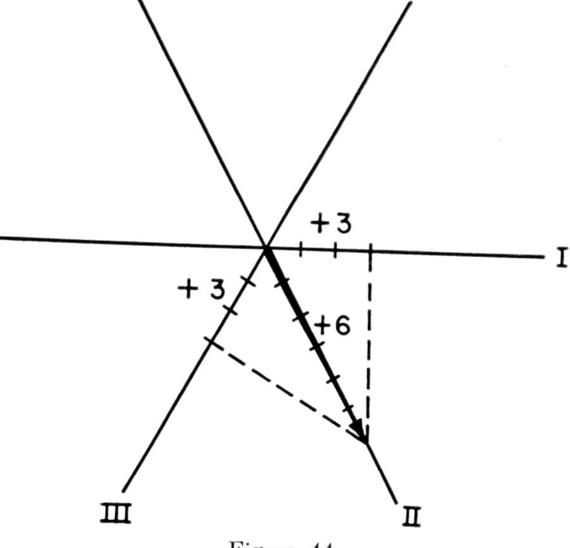

Figure 44.

and 5 units in Lead III. The perpendicular from Lead I to the tip of the vector will fall at zero on Lead I. Such a vector will record no potential in Lead I. This satisfies Einthoven's Law as well as the Law of Parallelograms. Another important vector principle is illustrated. *When the axis of a vector is 90° away from the lead axis, no potential is measured by that lead. Such a lead is called a diphasic or isoelectric lead* (Fig. 45).

A vector with an axis of +30° (perpendicular to Lead II), records no potential in Lead III. A vector with an axis of −30° (perpendicular to

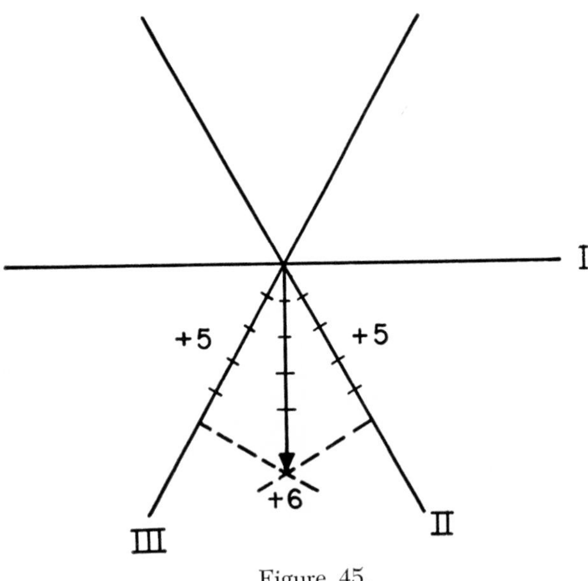

Figure 45.

Lead II) records no potential in Lead II. The axis of a vector can be determined by inspection alone, whenever one of the three leads is diphasic or isoelectric.

THE V LEAD

A bipolar lead measures the potential difference between two points. Utilizing the three standard leads, it is impossible to record the potential received at any one point due to the influence of the other electrode. Wilson devised a method of eliminating the mathematical value of the negative electrode. This was accomplished by attaching the negative terminal of the conductor to the right arm, left arm, and left leg. The value received at the negative pole would theoretically be zero (Fig. 46).

The principle of zero potential at the negative electrode is illustrated as follows: Assume a vector with a magnitude of +10 and an axis of +90°. The potential received by a negative electrode Vf would be −10, by the negative

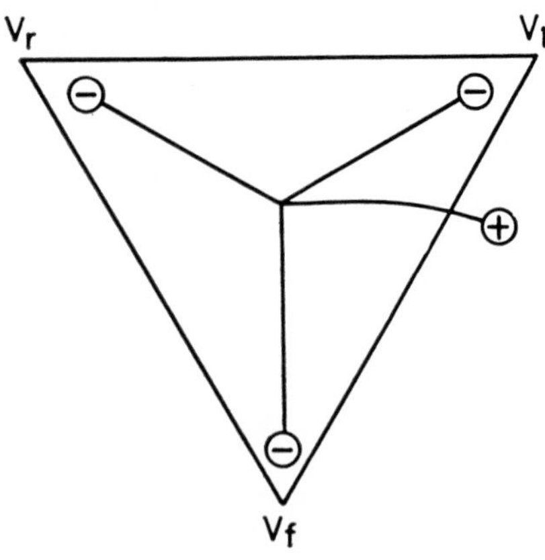

Figure 46.

electrode Vr, −5, by the negative electrode Vl, −5. By algebraic addition, − (+10) − (−5) − (−5) = −10 +5 +5 = 0. The positive electrode could then be placed at any point and measure only the potential received at that point. Such a lead is called a V lead, or an exploring electrode.

THE UNIPOLAR TRIAXIAL REFERENCE SYSTEM

Placing an exploring electrode (V lead) on the right arm, left arm, and left leg creates leads Vr, Vl, and Vf. The axis of Lead Vr may be depicted by drawing a line from the right shoulder to the center of zero potential. Lead Vl has an axis from the left shoulder to the zero center. Lead Vf has an axis from the pubis to the center of zero potential. Vr, Vl, and Vf bisect each angle of Einthoven's triangle. The negative terminal is the same for each lead, and equivalent to zero. This point may be considered as the point of origin for the three leads. If the axis of each lead is extended beyond its point of origin, another Triaxial Reference System is formed with 60° between each axis (Fig. 47).

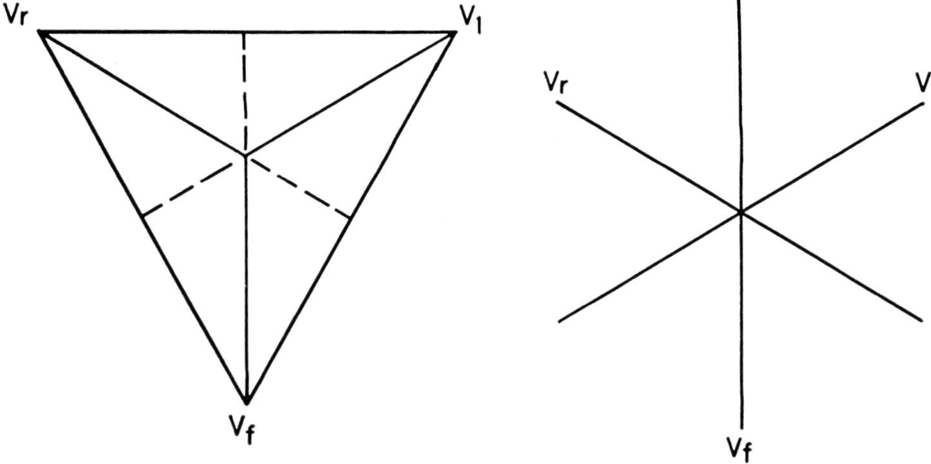

Figure 47.

The unipolar limb leads also bear a mathematical relation to one another. This may be expressed: Vr + Vl + Vf = 0. If a force with an axis of +90° and a magnitude of 6 units is measured by all three leads, Lead Vf = +6, Vr is –3, Vl is –3. This may be expressed: +6 –3 –3 = 0.

HEXAXIAL REFERENCE SYSTEM

The Unipolar Triaxial Reference System is rotated 30° away from the Bipolar Triaxial Reference System. By superimposing the point of origin for both Triaxial Reference Systems, a Hexaxial Reference System is formed (Fig. 48). The positive electrode of Vr has an axis of –150°, Vl –30° and Vf +90°.

AUGMENTED UNIPOLAR LEADS

Because the influence of the negative pole is removed, the amplitude of the unipolar leads is only half that obtained by the bipolar limb leads. Goldberger amplified (augmented) the potential by removing the negative electrode from Vl when the positive electrode was on the left arm, and in a like manner on the other extremities. To indicate this augmentation, the prefix *"a"* was added before the symbol of each lead (aVr, aVl, aVf). Even with augmentation the relative deflection obtained in the augmented limb leads is equivalent to only 86% of the value measured by the bipolar leads.

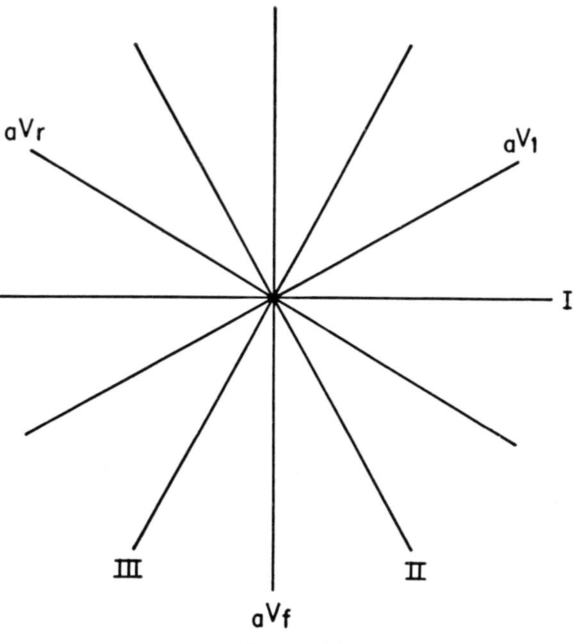

Figure 48.

AXIS BY INSPECTION

If the unipolar limb leads were equivalent to the bipolar limb leads, the lead with the most positive deflection would be most nearly parallel to the vector axis. Regardless of the relative sensitivity of each lead no potential will be registered at a point perpendicular to the vector (Fig. 49). This principle enables one to tell by simple inspection of the six limb leads the axis of any force. If no potential is recorded in Lead

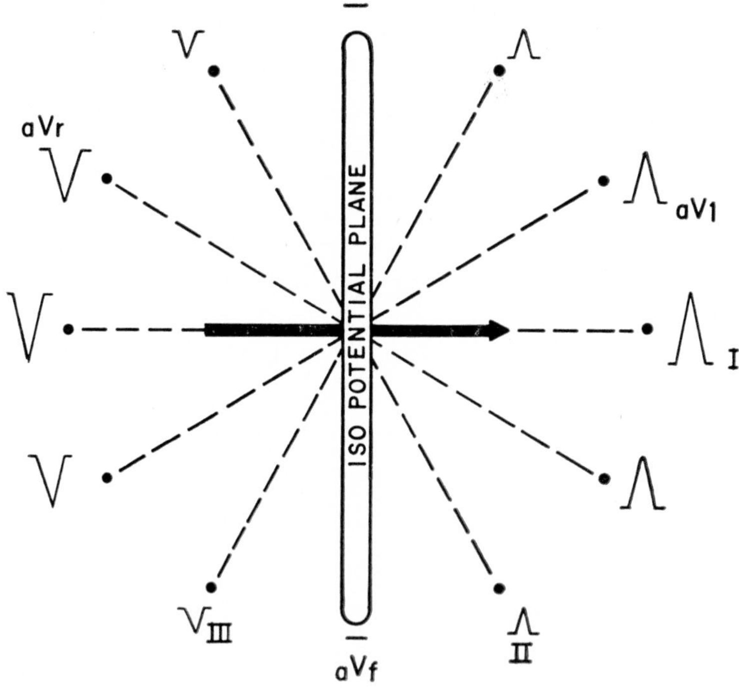

Figure 49

aVl (axis −30°), the axis of the vector is +60° (90° away from aVl). In this event, Lead II will record a strongly positive force. The vector axis could have been −120°. In the latter case, the force would be directed away from the positive terminal of Lead II and the complex in Lead II would be negative (Fig. 50).

To summarize the above discussion, the following rules may be formulated:

1) When a vector force faces a positive electrode, a positive wave is recorded.

2) When a vector force is going away from the positive electrode (towards the negative electrode) a negative wave is recorded.

3) The lead axis most closely parallel to the axis of a vector will record the greatest negative, or greatest positive, deflection (allowing for differences in value of the augmented unipolar and bipolar leads).

4) Ninety degrees away from a vector, the mathematical value of the potential measured equals zero (this perpendicular plane is called an isopotential plane).

5) Utilizing the Hexaxial Reference System,

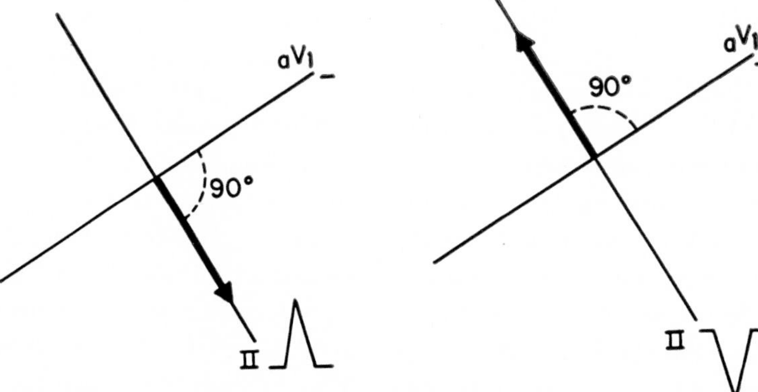

Figure 50.

one may determine the axis of any vector by the following steps:

a) Select the lead recording an isoelectric (mathematical zero) complex. The axis of this lead is the axis of the isopotential plane for the vector.

b) Ninety degrees away from the isopotential plane is the direction of the vector. If the lead that is parallel with the direction of the vector records a negative wave, the axis of the vector is 180° away from the positive terminal of that lead.

When no isoelectric complex is recorded in any lead, the isopotential plane of the force can still be determined. This is done by noting the point on the Hexaxial Reference System where the recorded complexes change from positive to negative. If aVl records a negative complex, and Lead I records a positive value, the isopotential plane is between their lead axes (between –30° and 0°). One can arbitrarily locate the isopotential plane at –15°. Ninety degrees away from –15° would be +75° (Fig. 51). By using this method the axis of a vector can be determined within 5° to 10° of its true axis.

A vector with an axis between +30° and +60° will record positive values in all leads except Lead aVr. The axis of the vector can be deduced. A vector of +30° records an isoelectric value in Lead III, therefore, the vector must have an axis of more than +30°. A vector of +60° records an isoelectric value in Lead aVl, therefore, the axis must be less than +60°. Whenever all leads, except aVr, record a positive value, the vector must be between +30° and +60° (Fig. 52).

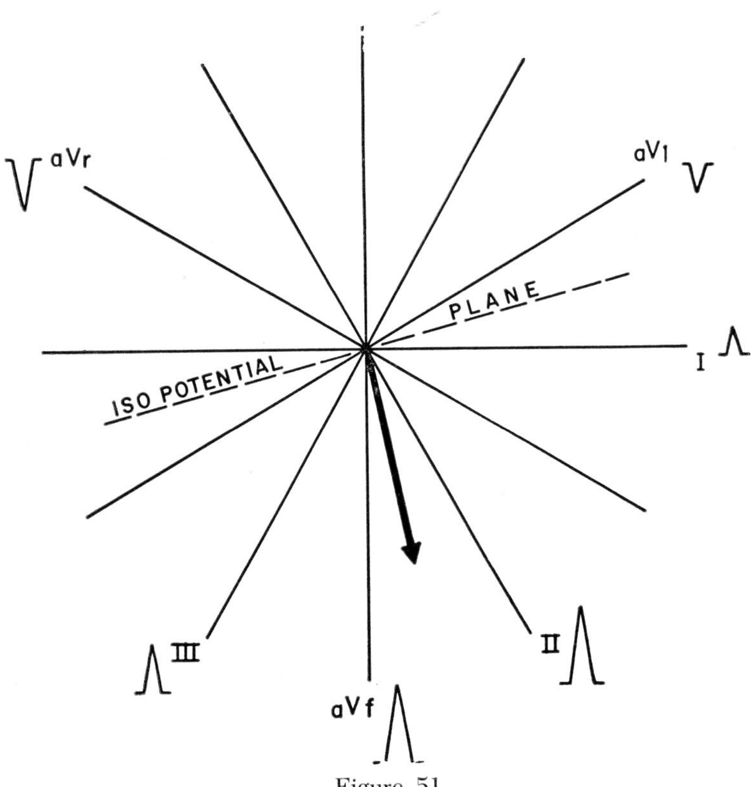

Figure 51.

THE FRONTAL PLANE

The Hexaxial Reference System describes a plane around the body. This plane is flat like a sheet of paper, and has no depth. If a vector is acting only in this plane, its total value can be measured by the Hexaxial Reference System. The vector forces originating from the heart are also directed either anteriorly or posteriorly. The six limb leads measure only the projection of the spatial vector on the frontal plane. The

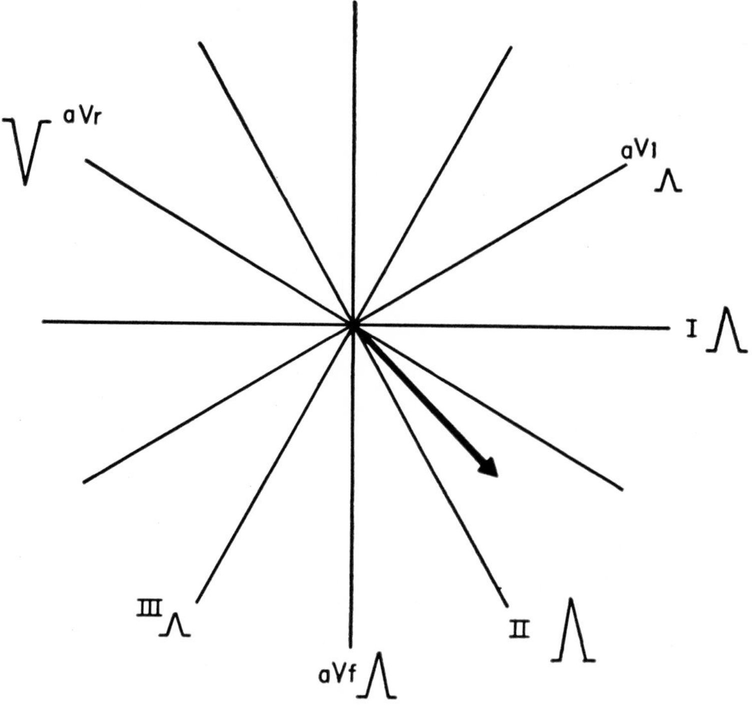

Figure 52.

more anterior or posterior the vector, the less will be its magnitude of projection on the frontal plane. The two perpendicular coordinates (X and Y) of the frontal plane are lead axis I and lead axis aVf.

THE TRANSVERSE PLANE

The projection of a cardiac vector on the transverse plane is measured by the V leads. This plane may be described as a cross section through the chest. The transverse plane consists of two perpendicular coordinates. One coordinate is parallel with Lead I and is the X coordinate. The other coordinate is the Z coordinate, measuring the anterior posterior component of the vector.

The V lead electrodes used to measure precordial potential, are, as described previously, for an exploring electrode. The location for each V lead comprising the transverse plane is at a specific anatomic site. The usual leads taken are at six sites, around a little more than a quarter of the circumference of the chest. Their locations are as follows (Fig. 53):

V1 Fourth interspace to the right of the sternum.
V2 Fourth interspace to the left of the sternum.
V3 Halfway between V2 and V4.
V4 Fifth interspace left midclavicular line.

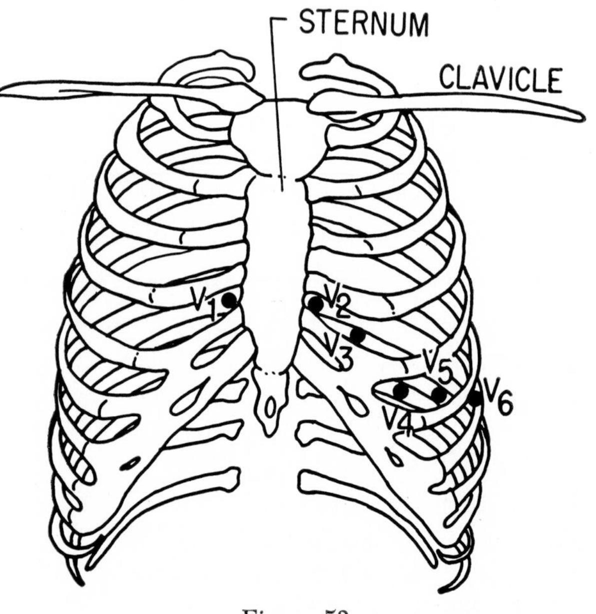

Figure 53.

V5 The same horizontal plane as V4 and in the anterior axillary line.
V6 The same horizontal plane as V4 and V5 in the mid axillary line.

Occasionally it is desirable to measure potential at additional areas. Right precordial leads may be used. These leads are called VR leads. They are in exactly similar locations as the usual left chest leads only on the right side. V1R is the same as V2 position. V2R is the same as V1. V3R is comparable to V3 position only on the right chest rather than the left (Fig. 54).

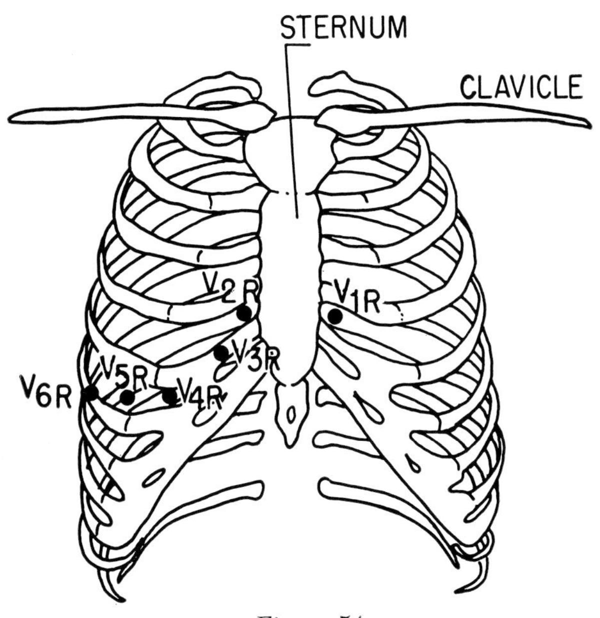

Figure 54.

When the posterior axillary line position is utilized, it is called V7. A point at the level of V6 and in the left tip of the scapula is utilized for V8. Just to the left of the spine on the same level, is position V9.

The anterior precordial leads are not usually considered "remote." Their location is not sufficiently distant from the heart for a "remote" electrode. Their proximity results in discrepancies in amplitude. Nevertheless, when the precordial electrode is located in the positive electrical field, positive force will be recorded and when in the negative electrical field, a negative wave is recorded. This enables one to locate the isopotential plane for a cardiac vector. The vector force between the two electrical fields is perpendicular to the isopotential plane. Locating the vector in the transverse plane is possible by first locating the isopotential plane on the chest.

When the V lead position is sufficiently distant from the heart to be considered "remote" the potential at its location is expressed simply as $\frac{3}{r^2}$. It differs from the previously described bipolar leads in that no angle exists between the lead axis and the radius distance as they are one and the same.

The proximity of the precordial leads to the zero center exaggerates small variations in the location of the center. While it is recognized that the zero center has individual variations, its location can be approximated. Most authorities agree that it lies anteriorly to the anatomic center of the thorax. It is convenient and practical to consider its location at a point between V6 and V6R at the level of the fourth intercostal space, and just to the left of the sternum. The zero center can then be located as the point where Leads I, aVf and V2 intersect and are mutually perpendicular. These three leads form three mutually perpendicular coordinates (X, Y, Z).

All V leads have the same theoretic negative pole, the zero center. They comprise an axis system for the transverse plane. The angle between each V lead axis will have individual variations but an approximation can be utilized.

Because the zero center is displaced anteriorly it is considered on a plane between V6 and V6R positions (a plane between the mid axillary lines). Often V6 may be just a little posterior to the true plane of zero potential, however, V6 position is more nearly correct than V5, which is usually anterior to the zero center plane.

V2 is one of the perpendicular coordinates and 90° away from V6. Lead axis V3 forms an angle of 20° with lead axis V2. Lead axis V4 forms a 40° angle with lead axis V2. Lead axis V5 forms a 70° angle with V2. The axis of Lead I is parallel to the axis of Lead V6. As a reference system in the transverse plane, it is convenient to call V6 zero degrees. Every point posterior to V6 is considered positive. The transverse plane axes can be located as follows (Fig. 55):

V1 = –110°
V2 = – 90°
V3 = – 70°
V4 = – 50°
V5 = – 20°
V6 = 0°

transverse plane by the magnitude along the X axis. The product is the magnitude of the vector in the transverse plane.

THE TWELVE LEAD SPATIAL REFERENCE SYSTEM

If one superimposed the point of origin for both the Hexaxial Reference System and the Transverse Reference System, a Spatial Reference System is formed (Fig. 57).

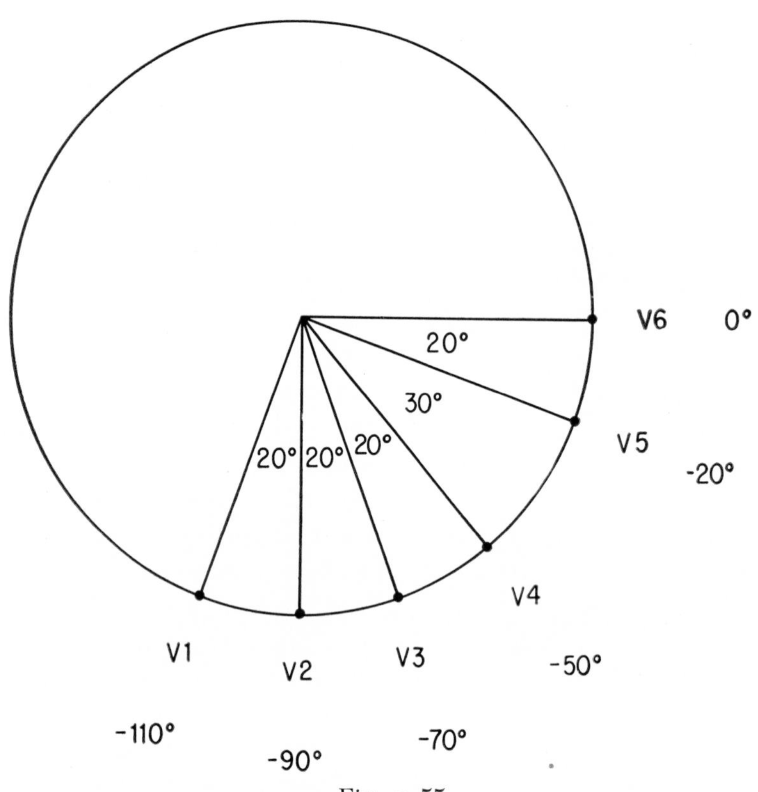

Figure 55.

The magnitude of the vector projected on the transverse plane can be determined by the following steps (Fig. 56):

1) Locate the isopotential point, e.g., V3 at –70°.

2) The transverse vector is projected 90° away from that point, i.e., +20°. (Twenty degrees is the angle between the vector and the X coordinate, or Leads I and V6.)

3) Measure the mean value of the vector on its X axis in the frontal plane (Lead I).

4) Multiply the cosine of the angle in the

As previously discussed, the magnitude of the spatial vector measured by the X and Y coordinates can be determined from the frontal plane. The magnitude projected on Z coordinate can be determined by multiplying the sine of the angle in the transverse plane by the magnitude along X coordinate (sine of angle a = cosine of angle b) (Fig. 58). The magnitude of the spatial vector can be calculated. It has been demonstrated that the X, Y, Z coordinate values can be obtained. The magnitude of the spatial vector measured by the coordinates is determined

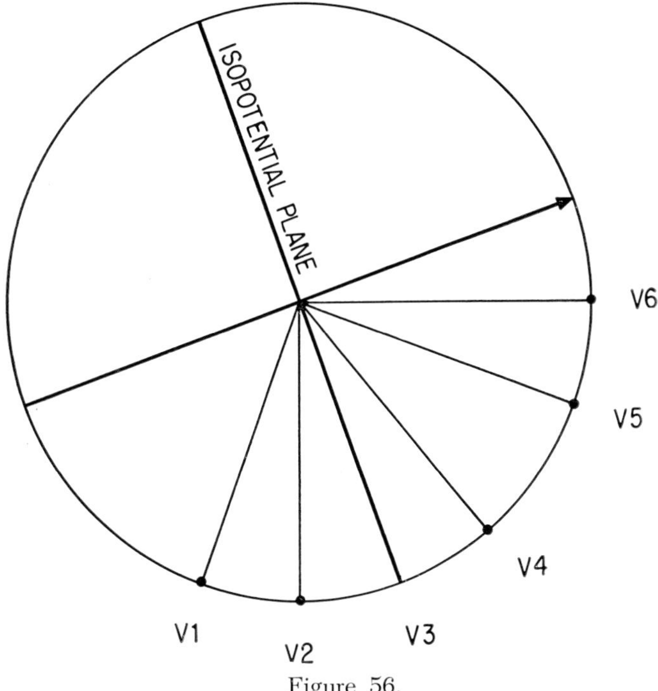

Figure 56.

by utilizing the rule of squared coordinates. The magnitude of any force squared, equals the sum of the squares of its projection on each of its coordinates.

Lead measurement of spatial vector magnitude $= X^2 + Y^2 + Z^2$.

The calculations of magnitude given above are based on Lead I measurement of magnitude. Lead I was shown to measure $3L/r^3$ of a vector. Thus the relative magnitude of the spatial vector at its point of origin in the volume conductor is: lead measurement of spatial vector magni-

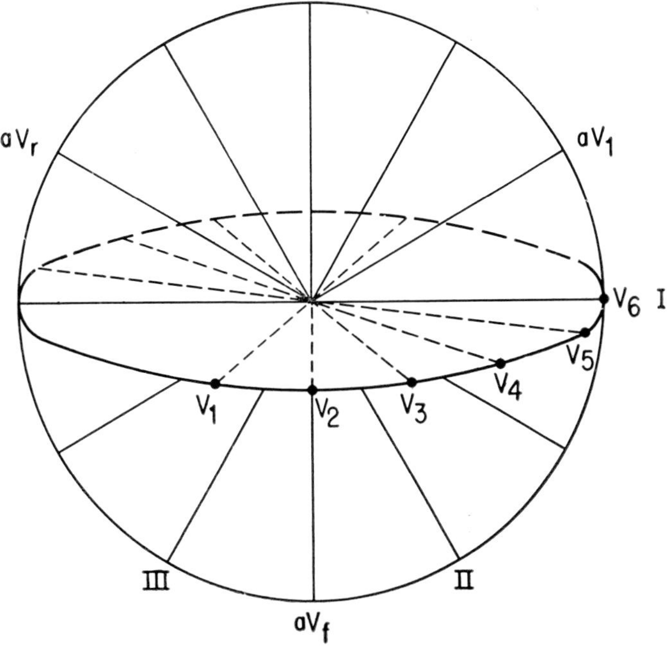

Figure 57.

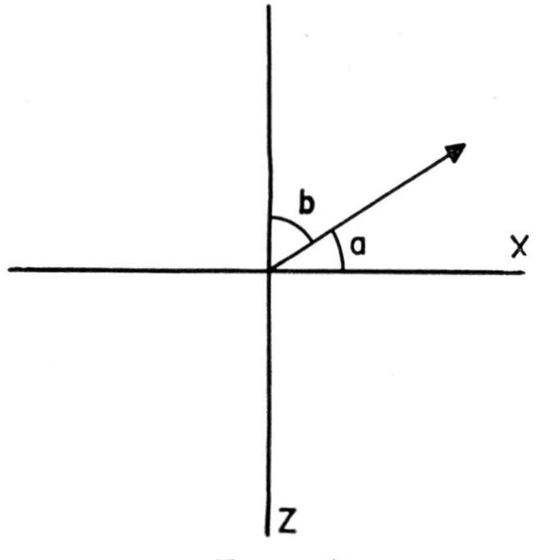

Figure 58.

tude times $\frac{r^3}{3L}$, where r is the radius and L is the length of Lead I.

SAGITTAL PLANE

The sagittal plane is comprised of the Y and Z coordinates, or aVf and V2. It is the profile of the body (Fig. 59). The direction and magnitude of any vector can be determined in the sagittal plane by using the values obtained for Y and Z coordinates in the frontal and transverse planes.

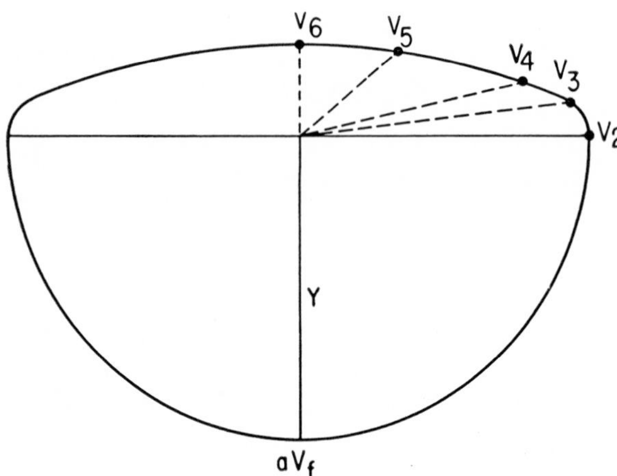

Figure 59. A right profile of the Sagittal Plane.

EFFECTS OF ECCENTRIC ZERO CENTER

The simplified presentation of the centric dipole concept given above is not exactly correct. The zero center is eccentric in location and the lead lengths are not equal. The routine ECG finds its greatest application in the measurement of duration, sequence of events, and relative direction of one spatial vector to another. Errors in directional measurements are largely the same for all vectors in the same individual, thus measuring the spatial angle between two vectors is practical. The normal values obtained for ECG measurements are based on the centric dipole concept and comparisons cannot be made with any other concept until other normal values are obtained. The errors imposed by the assumption of a centric dipole should be understood to evaluate the unusual circumstance and to comprehend the advances occurring in this rapidly changing field.

An example of the errors imposed can be obtained from considering the fundamentals of Lead I (Fig. 60). Due to eccentric location of the zero center, Lead I is not a balanced bipolar lead. The leftward position of the zero center permits the vertical and sagittal component of the spatial vector to influence the lead measurement. The vertical component directed towards the foot has a negative influence on the lead measurement. The magnitude of the influence depends upon the magnitude of the vertical component and the degree of eccentricity.

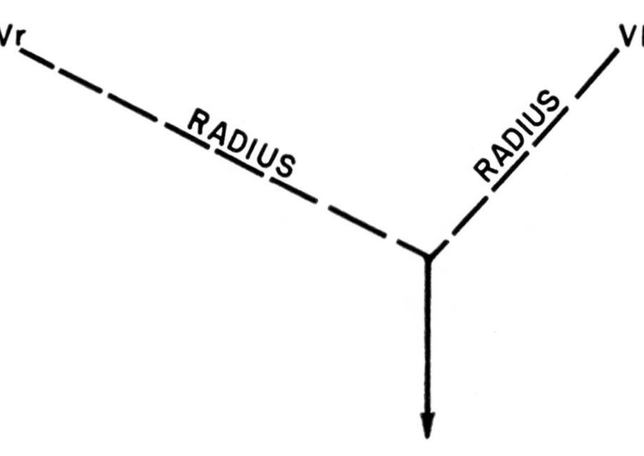

Figure 60.

It is clear that if Lead I is to be used to measure only the X component of a spatial force it must be a true bipolar lead. Similar effects occur in Lead II and Lead III. Usually, elec-

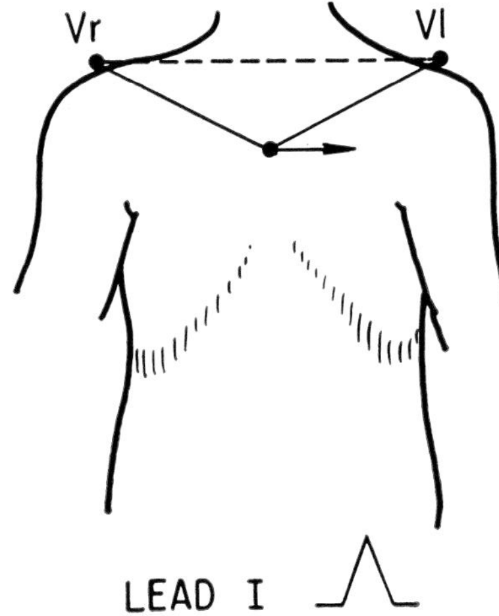

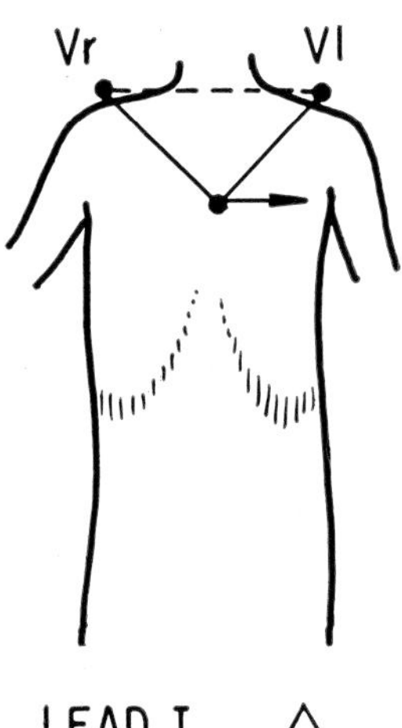

Figure 61.

trode Vl records a much larger negative influence from the vertical vector than Vr because the radius distance of Vl is shorter and the obtuse angle is greater. Eccentricity can cause an initial negative wave in Lead I. Such factors are responsible for many ECG patterns that have been ascribed to septal depolarization and other anatomic correlations. No attempt at anatomic correlation should be made unless the leads used are true equal bipolar leads or true unipolar leads.

The V leads are also effected by eccentricity of the zero center. The value measured at the negative electrode is not really zero in these circumstances and the positive V lead electrode does not represent the point potential at its location but the difference in potential at that point and the value of the negative terminal.

LEAD LENGTH AND VECTOR AXIS

Lead length depends upon the physical contour and shape of the human body. The individual with a short, squat chest has a long axis for Lead I, and records a large potential value for the transverse (X) component. The individual with the long, narrow chest has a relatively short Lead I axis and records a small potential value for the transverse component. The latter ECG records a more vertical vector and the former a more horizontal vector, even though the actual direction of the spatial vector may be identical in both individuals. Thus, the vertical vector and transverse vector, as described by the usual ECG is also an expression of the shape of the volume conductor (Fig. 61).

The principle of lead length is clearly seen from the formula for magnitude: Lead I = X component magnitude times $\frac{3L}{r^3}$. When the X component magnitude and the radius are constant the magnitude measured by Lead I is proportional to the lead length.

LIMITATIONS OF ROUTINE ELECTROCARDIOGRAPHY

The limitations in the use of the routine ECG may be summed up as follows:

1) Variations due to eccentric dipole position.

2) Variations in lead length due to physical shape of the volume conductor.

3) Variations imposed by nonhomogeneity of the volume conductor.

4) Inability to measure the magnitude of component forces and their duration from a coordinate graph, as these are measured only from the peripheral arc of the rotating central resultant.

5) When using the direct writing instrument sensitivity to more rapid events is lost.

These criticisms do not mean that routine electrocardiography is not a useful and valid tool, but serve to point up that its full application has not been realized. Direct writing instruments offer the distinct advantage of a practical bedside or field instrument, but they are not adequate for study of more complicated problems or for investigation. The problems associated with the first four limitations given above are somewhat mitigated by the use of a less sensitive instrument.

The routine ECG should be used to measure duration, sequence and relative direction of spatial forces. It may be used in a somewhat more coarse fashion for magnitude measurements.

VII

The Normal Electrocardiogram

THE P WAVE

THE FIRST EVENT of the normal cardiac cycle is atrial excitation, creating a P loop. The projection of this event on a lead axis creates the initial wave called the P wave. The character of the P wave in a given lead depends upon the P loop and the lead axis (Fig. 62). Usually the P loop is located between zero and ninety degrees (between the axis of Lead I and aVf). The P loop is directed towards the positive pole of Lead I and II creating a positive P wave in those leads. If the force is directed leftward parallel to Lead I, the P wave will be positive in aVl and negative in Lead III. A P loop directed downward towards aVf will cause a negative P wave in aVl. Often there is a biphasic P wave at V1 or V2 with an initial positive displacement and terminal negative component. The force of atrial excitation is above the electrode at its onset and below it as well as posterior, terminally. By more remote electrodes (V9) it is seen that the P loop is chiefly posterior. Variations in configuration are numerous.

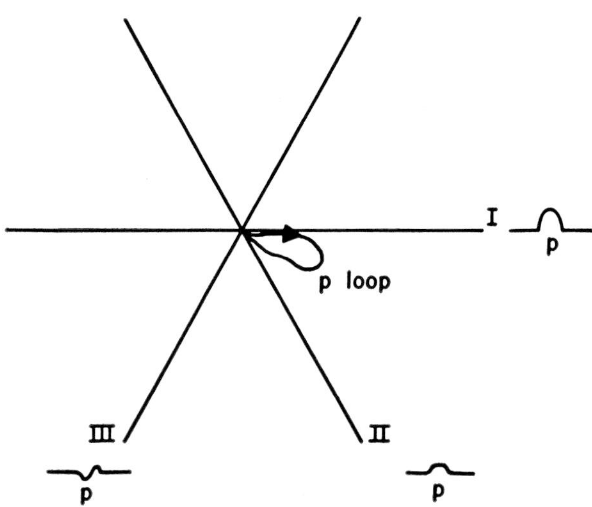

Figure 62.

The duration of the P wave reflects the time required for atrial excitation. Atrial excitation can require no less time than the longest P wave duration in any lead. A more precise measurement requires simultaneous recording of three mutually perpendicular leads. *Normally the P wave duration does not exceed 0.12 sec.* In general, the greater the P wave duration, the greater is the surface area of the atria.

The amplitude of the P wave is dependent upon the effective area of the wave front of excitation. In turn, this is dependent upon wall thickness. Amplitude measurements are fraught with pitfalls due to such factors as conduction and distance. For this reason P wave amplitude is best evaluated by comparing its amplitude to other events, ventricular excitation and recovery. *A very general rule is to regard any P wave of 3 mm. amplitude as unusually large,* then compare to see if all the events are increased in amplitude or only the P wave.

THE PR INTERVAL

The interval between the onset of the P wave and the onset of ventricular excitation is called the PR interval (Fig. 63). It measures the time between the onset of atrial excitation and beginning of ventricular excitation. It includes the time required for atrial excitation (P wave) and the time required for transmission of the impulse through the AV node and its ramifications to ventricular muscle reception areas. The latter is represented by a nearly isoelectric interval

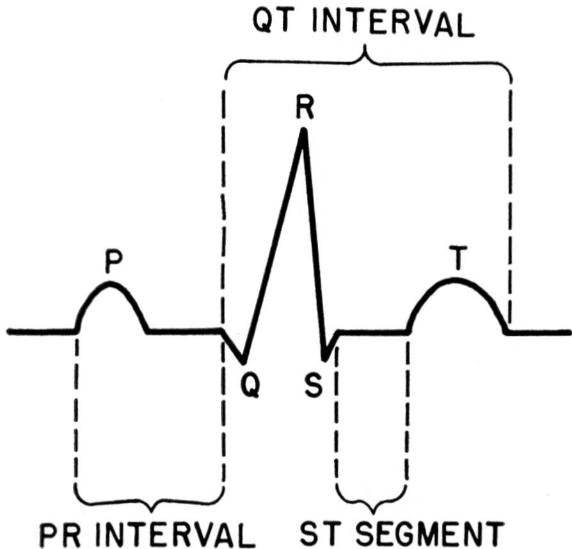

Figure 63.

between the P wave and the onset of ventricular excitation (approximately .06 to .08 sec.).

The PR interval varies with age and heart rate. In the adult with a heart rate of 80 per minute, *the PR interval should not exceed .20 sec.* A PR interval of .20 sec. at a heart rate of 90 per minute is abnormal. A PR interval of .10 sec. or less is also abnormal indicating a change in the usual order of excitation.

Care should be taken to measure the PR interval in a lead with the longest QRS duration and a sharply defined P wave of greatest duration. Otherwise the measurement may not reflect the true time required for transmission of the impulse from the SA node to ventricular muscle. Simultaneous leads obviate this difficulty.

THE QRS COMPLEX

Configuration. The forces of ventricular excitation, graphed on a lead axis are called the QRS complex. By convention, when the initial wave is negative it is called a Q wave. The first positive wave is called an R wave. The first negative wave (below the base line) following a positive wave is called an S wave. A positive wave following an S wave is called an R′ wave. Thus the initial events may create a Q wave in one lead and an R wave in another lead. A deflection of an R wave toward the base line followed by a secondary increase in amplitude is not an S wave. Such a change is notching of the R wave.

If a wave is of small amplitude, it is often printed in small letters and if large, printed in capital letters. A small q wave, a large R wave, and a small s wave is written qRs. When the entire QRS complex is a large negative deflection, it may be called a QS deflection.

The QRS configuration in any lead depends upon the relation of the lead axis to the spatial pathway of ventricular excitation. Consider a simple pathway directed anteriorly to the left and downward, then returning posteriorly to the right and to the center of origin (Fig. 64).

Lead I will have an initial R wave. The max-

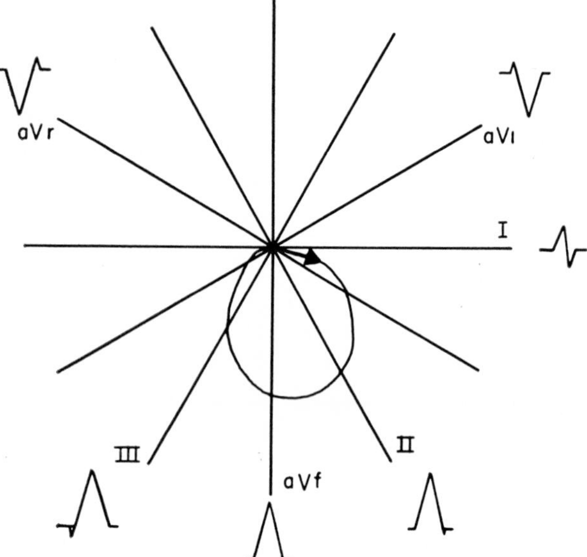

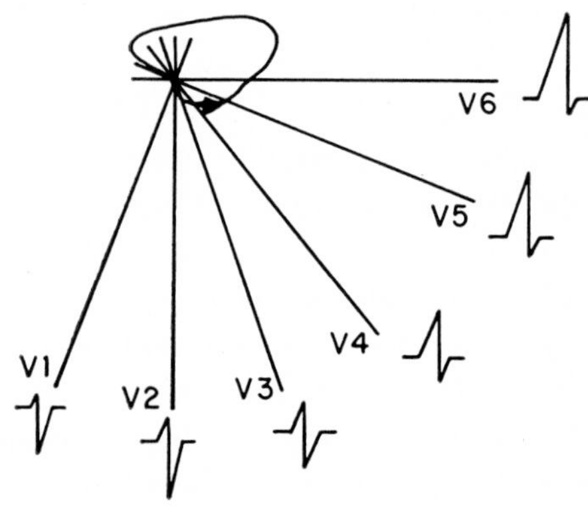

Figure 64.

imum height of the R wave corresponds in time to the most leftward point on the QRS pathway. Its amplitude is proportional to the X component of the instantaneous vector occurring at that time interval. The R wave diminishes in amplitude as the pathway becomes more perpendicular to the axis of Lead I. The S wave begins as the pathway moves more than 90° away from the positive terminal of Lead I. The most negative point of the S wave corresponds to the time the spatial pathway reaches its most rightward point. The S wave diminishes as the pathway returns to the center of origin.

By remembering the lead axis, the instantaneous vectors at each time interval can be graphed as a coordinate graph. Thus the QRS complex can be built for each lead.

The maximum left and right course is depicted by Lead I. The maximum downward point is the height of the R wave in aVf. By correlating simultaneous leads, the spatial pathway can be reconstructed in a general manner from the QRS complexes. To accurately reflect the spatial pathway, other factors such as lead length, radius distance and zero center location must be considered.

The precordial leads, in a somewhat more general fashion, correspond to the spatial QRS pathway. The time of the height of the R wave in V2 corresponds to the time of the maximum anterior course of the QRS pathway. The time and magnitude of the height of the R wave increases at more leftward positions. This reflects more of the spatial pathway being in the positive zone of the lead axis. The R wave in Lead V6 records the maximum leftward course of the QRS pathway. It begins to lose amplitude as the pathway loses its leftward location. The maximum posterior course of the loop corresponds to the maximum negative point (S wave) in V2.

The Intrinsicoid Deflection. An electrode placed directly on a segment of heart muscle will record a positive wave as excitation moves outward to the surface. When excitation reaches the surface, a deflection below the base line occurs instantly. This deflection is called *the intrinsic deflection.* The time between the onset of excitation and the onset of the intrinsic deflection is an index of the thickness of the muscle directly beneath the electrode. The time of onset of the intrinsic deflection is delayed when the muscle is abnormally thick.

The principle of the intrinsic deflection is indeed valid for electrodes placed directly on the heart. However, electrodes from the body surface behave differently and are in certain respects remote, reflecting the action of the heart muscle as a whole. One school of investigators chose to consider the electrodes on the chest as behaving like they were influenced chiefly by the segment of muscle beneath them. Thus the downward deflection at any electrode position represented the thickness of the muscle mass beneath. This deflection being intrinsic like it was called *the intrinsicoid deflection* (coid means like).

The "intrinsicoid" deflection at V1 has been called an index of right ventricular wall thickness and its upper limit of normal given as .035 sec. The "intrinsicoid" deflection at V6 has been called an index of left ventricular wall thickness with a normal valve up to .045 sec. The times are correctly measured as the onset of the deflection, i.e. the end of the peak of the R wave.*

In practical application I have found these measurements of little value. When they are truly abnormal there is no difficulty in diagnosing the disorder without this determination. Moreover the chest electrodes are markedly influenced by the entire heart. The time of the R wave peak in V2 corresponds to the time of the most anterior course of spatial QRS pathway, and is exactly equivalent to the time of the depth of the Q wave from an electrode directly opposite V2 on the back (Fig. 65). Thus the time interval is the same whether the electrode is on the front of the chest over the right ventricle or over the back over the left ventricle.

The peak of the S wave in V2 corresponds to the most posterior course of the spatial pathway.

---

*This was originally defined for the intrinsic deflection measurements. Lewis, T., and Rothschild, M. A.: *Philos. Tr. R. Soc., London, 206 s.B*:181, 1915.

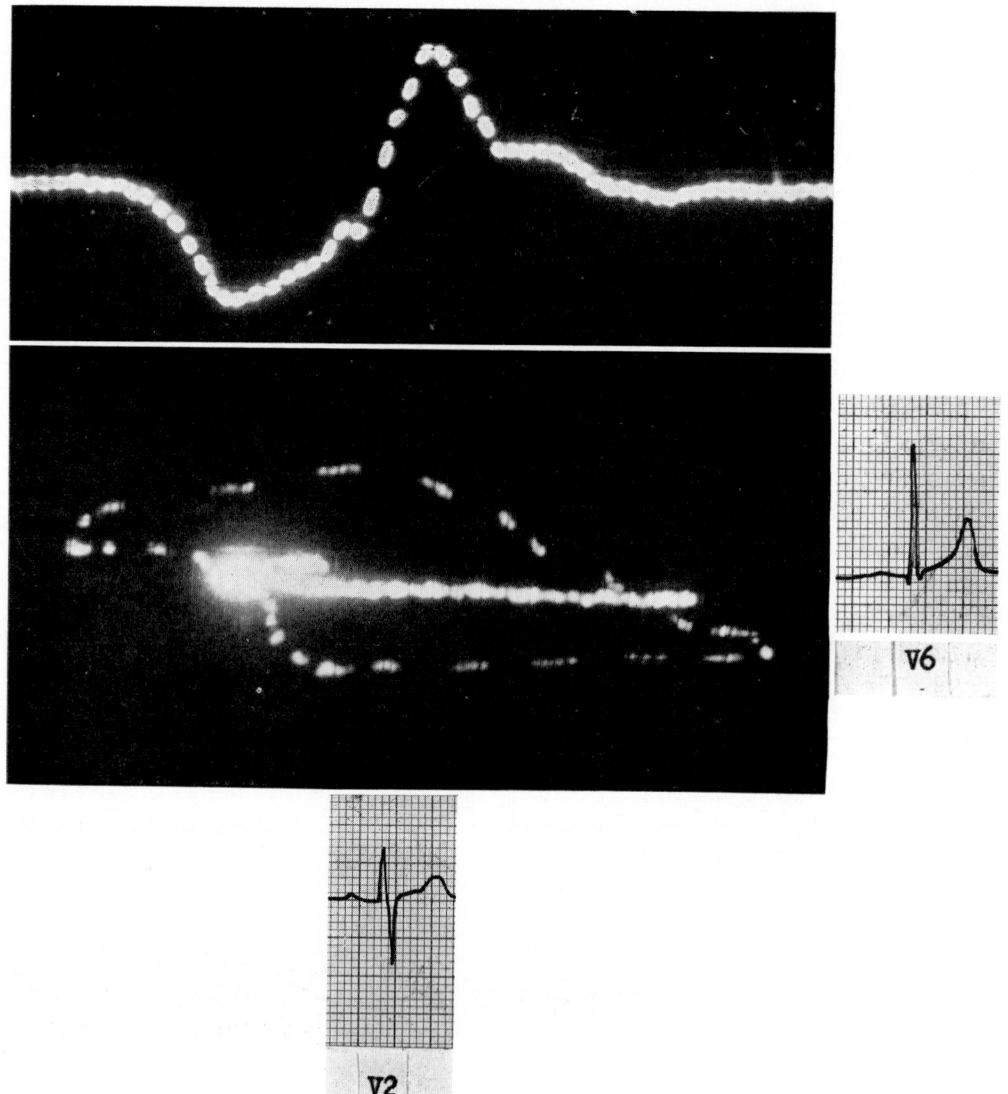

Figure 65. The anterior course of the QRS loop creates the initial Q wave in the V lead recorded from the back (top of figure) and an initial R wave in V2. As the loop reaches its most leftward point the height of the R wave in V6 is recorded. The terminal rightward course of the loop creates the terminal S wave at V6. Minor variations in initial Q waves and R waves are often due to placing the chest electrodes above or below the zero center. When this occurs they are no longer strictly recording the transverse plane.

The height of the R wave (intrinsicoid deflection) recorded by an electrode over the back occurs at the same time as the depth of the S wave at V2. Thus the "intrinsicoid" time of the left ventricle can be obtained from an electrode very proximal to the right ventricle. These observations are not compatible with the notion that chest electrodes behave like proximal electrodes in reflecting chiefly the activity of the muscle segment beneath them.

The intrinsicoid deflection at V6 actually measures the time of the most leftward course of the spatial pathway. Since the left ventricle is posterior and the septum is anterior much of left ventricular activation creates a posterior force occurring after the intrinsicoid deflection at V6. In the routine ECG left ventricular activation is often best represented by the S wave of V2.

Since the magnitude of the leftward course

normally increases as the right ventricular force declines, the maximum leftward magnitude occurs more closely to completion of right ventricular activity. For this reason the height of the R wave at V6 closely corresponds to the completion of right ventricular activation in the normal heart rather than the left ventricle. Indeed the time commonly given for completion of right ventricle activation (.03 to .04 sec.) will be found in the normal heart to be the time for the height of the R wave at V6.*

Duration. The QRS duration is measured to determine the length of time required for ventricular excitation. The longest QRS duration in any lead approximates the excitation interval. Lead V2 most often has the greatest QRS duration as the terminal activation of the left ventricle creates a posterior pathway. The ideal determination is made from three simultaneous mutually perpendicular leads. The QRS duration is an index of wall thickness. Since the wall becomes thicker from childhood to maturity, the QRS duration increases accordingly. *The normal QRS duration varies from .06 to .10 sec.*

Due to complications of the wave front at the base of the heart, discussed previously, the terminal QRS complex may be complicated or prolonged. This is particularly true in younger individuals. With maturity these variations are less common.

Amplitude. QRS amplitude is dependent upon the recording technique (lead lengths, electrode distances), density of charge across the wave front and the volume of the ventricles. The volume of the ventricles depends upon cardiac rate and phase of the respiratory cycle. Amplitude should be determined by using three perpendicular leads. A rough guide for QRS amplitude is the sum of the QRS amplitude in V2, aVf and V6. When this value exceeds 5.0 mv., increased amplitude should be considered. *Amplitude measurements of spatial forces require consideration of three perpendicular axes.*

Effects of Heart Rate. With a slow heart rate the stroke volume is increased. The increased volume is reflected in increased QRS amplitude. A rapid heart rate is associated with smaller QRS amplitude (Fig. 66).

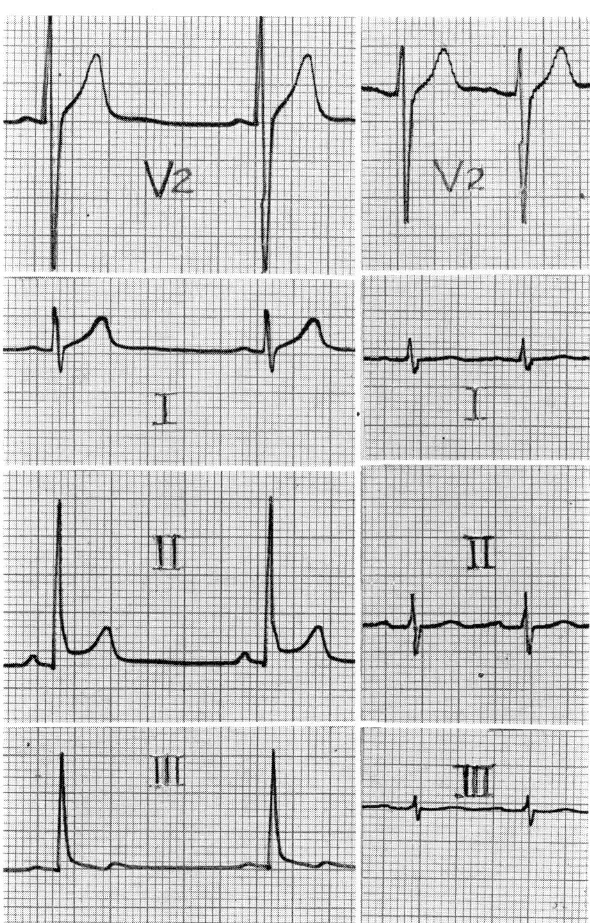

Figure 66. Note the difference in amplitude in two individuals of approximately the same age, health and size. Increased amplitude is seen with a rate of 55 per minute and low amplitude at a rate of 100 per minute.

Effects of Respiration. Respiration has a large effect on QRS amplitude and configuration. In the past these have been attributed to a simple change in heart position. An original observation indicates that the change is not a simple axis shift. In actuality the ECG is a sensitive measurement in the changes in left ventricular stroke volume. It is well known that inspiration

*The right ventricle begins activation .005 sec. after the left ventricle. By .02 sec. the confluent right ventricular cone is established. Muscle spread extends outward at 3 mm. each .01 sec. Allowing a wall thickness of 6 mm., the right ventricle will complete activation by .04 sec.

causes increased right ventricular stroke volume and diminishing left ventricular stroke volume.

During deep inspiration there is a progressive decrease in QRS amplitude in all leads. The initial .04 sec. period becomes more vertical with increased right ventricular volume. The terminal .04 sec. is diminished consistent with decreased left ventricular volume. A simple shift in axis requires that amplitude be increased in Lead II (Figs. 67 and 68). Holding the breath at deep inspiration causes slowing of the heart rate. In the vertical electrical axis it is noted that an S wave in Lead I disappears or is markedly diminished. A simple right axis shift would have the opposite effect increasing the S wave (Fig. 69).

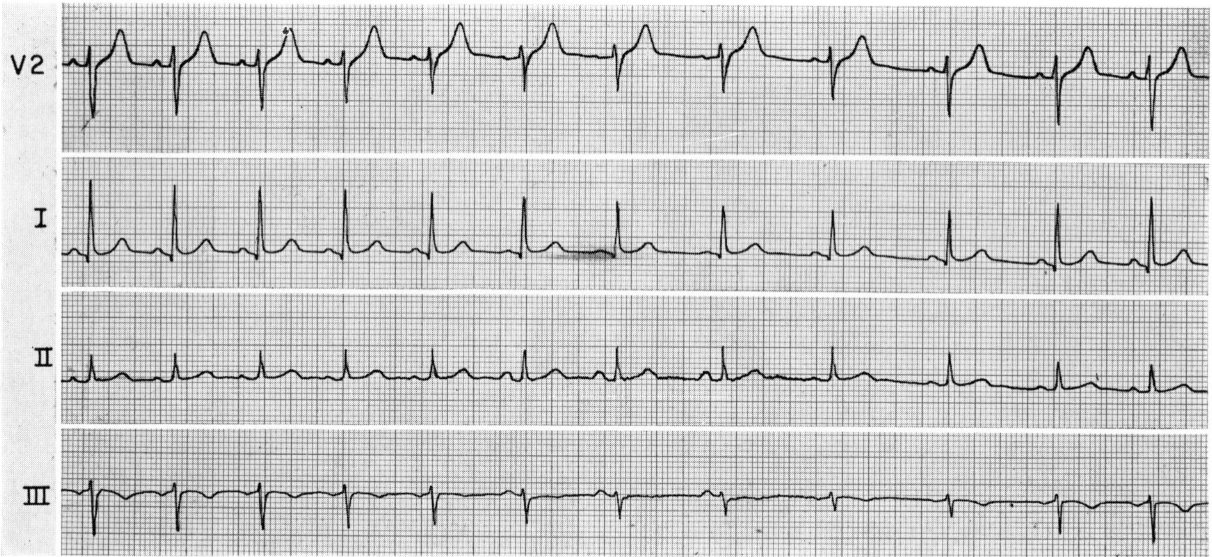

Figure 67. A simultaneous recording of four leads showing the decrease in QRS amplitude with inspiration and return to normal amplitude with expiration. Note the principal effect is on the terminal half of the QRS complex, not the first half. The last half of the QRS cycle is largely created by the left ventricle.

With inspiration, a late R wave in aVr will lose its prominence and a deep S wave may occur in aVl. This terminal change in the QRS events simply reflects a leftward (more vertical) shift of the terminal QRS forces. A shift in rightward axis with inspiration of necessity would increase the late R wave in aVr (Fig. 70).

A most striking example of the influence of respiration is noted in V2. The S wave behaves as a simple spirogram by its progressive diminution and increase in size (Fig. 71). This may be observed at quiet respiration in individuals with adequate stroke volume. It will be recalled that the S wave of V2 is chiefly due to the left ventricle.

The influence of respiration is further complicated by the increase in cardiac rate during inspiration. The increased rate can decrease diastolic filling with decreased volume causing diminished amplitude. However when the rate is stabilized with arrested inspiration, the pure effects of increased negative intrathoracic pressure is evident. When deep inspiration is held for some time the ECG begins to return toward normal. This reflects more or less complete filling of the pulmonary vascular bed, or in a sense a modified valsalva.

Change in conduction with lung inflation cannot be used as an explanation of diminished amplitude as the initial .04 sec. show increased amplitude. Moreover, V2 position is directly over the heart and not insulated by lung tissue even in full inspiration. The drop in QRS amplitude is also manifested in all leads when a premature nodal or atrial contraction occurs early enough to markedly diminish diastolic filling.

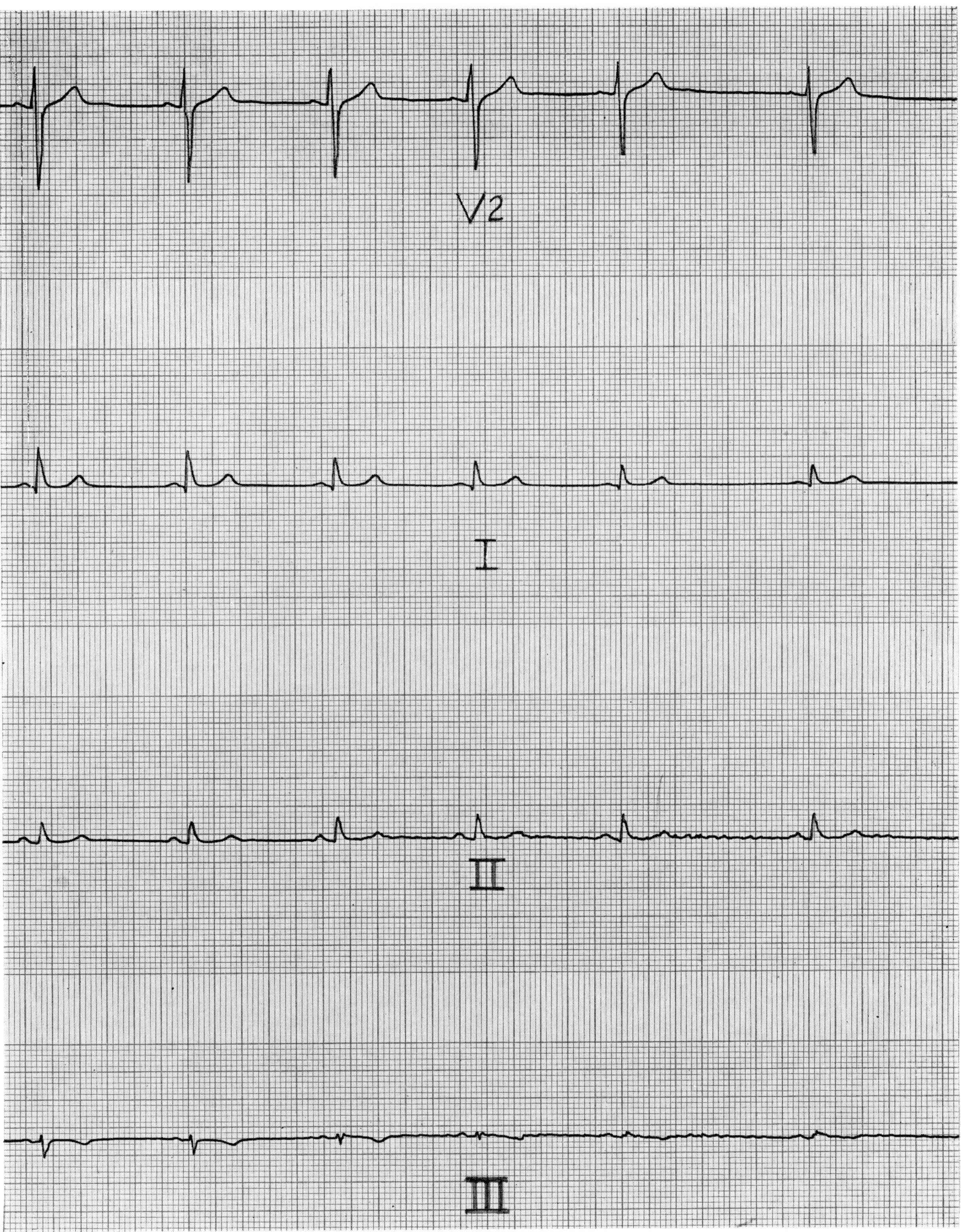

Figure 68. Another example of the overall change in QRS amplitude caused by inspiration. A simple anatomic change in cardiac position due to the lowering of the diaphragm should cause increased amplitude in Lead II as the electrical position becomes more vertical. This simply does not occur.

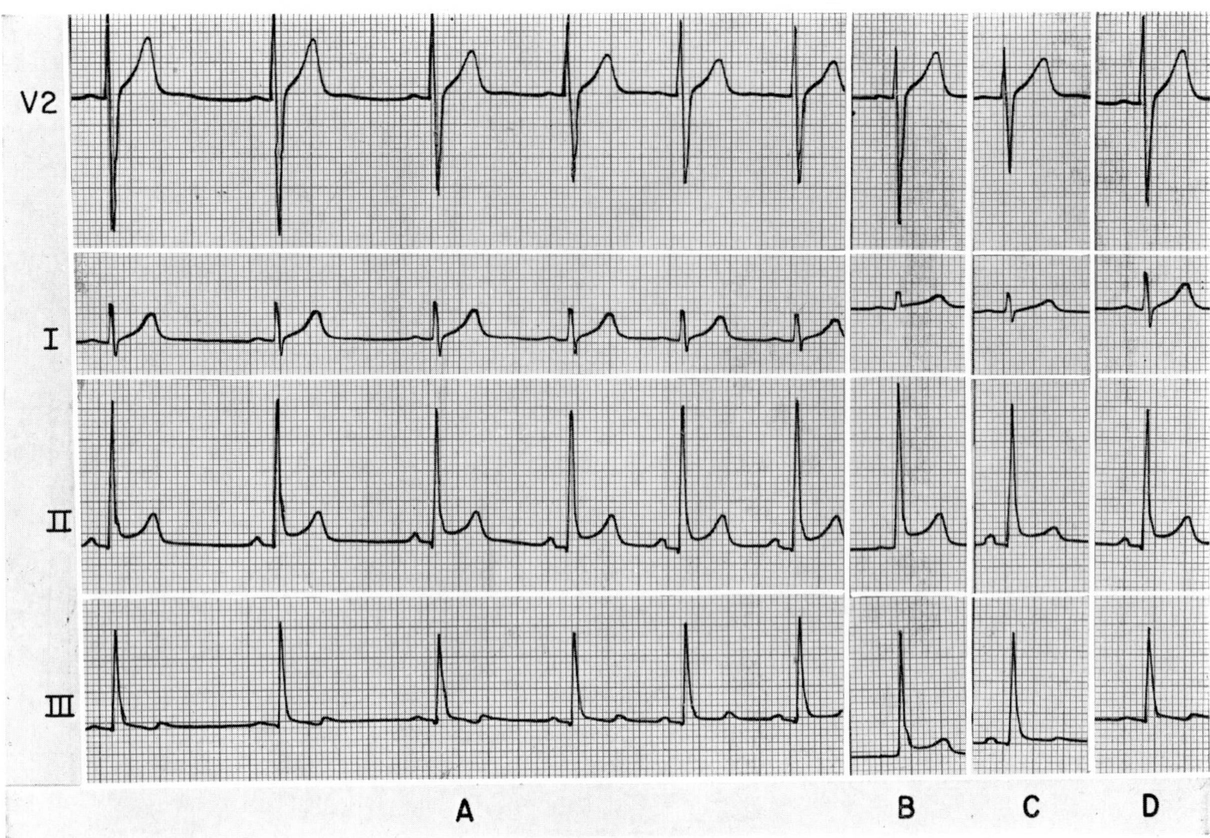

Figure 69. A) The inspiratory phase of the respiratory cycle with decreased amplitude of the S wave in V2. B) Holding the breath at the height of inspiration. Note the S wave in Lead I entirely disappears, completely contrary to a simple right axis shift. C) After holding the breath for 30 seconds at full inspiration the QRS amplitude increases, despite the fact that insulation and mechanical effects of lung inflation are at the maximum. D) On expiration about the fifth cycle later, the QRS amplitude is the same as at the onset of the maneuver.

This is not associated with respiration (Fig. 72). Also against the theory of insulation is increased P loop magnitude observed during inspiration and decreased P loop magnitude with expiration. Moreover insulation is theoretically greatest with deep inspiration and with prolonged held deep inspiration the ECG changes back toward normal.

The observation that the ECG can be used as an index of difference in right and left ventricular stroke volume creates a whole new avenue of investigation in electrocardiography including the possibilities of application to pulmonary function. It is interesting to note that the ballistocardiograph has long been touted as superior to the ECG because it could be correlated to stroke volume. Changes in the ballistocardiograph have been correlated to the respiratory cycle. The above observations indicate the ECG may be useful for this measurement.

Effects of Exercise. The usual response of the young lean individual to acute exercise is an increase in rate maintaining stroke volume. The QRS amplitude remains unchanged. There are a group of individuals that respond differently. Immediately after exercise they have a decrease in QRS amplitude associated with an increase in rate. As the rate slows the QRS amplitude returns to normal. Although the group observed to date is small it appears to be in those individuals who are overweight and do little physical exercise. One explanation for their decreased QRS amplitude is diminished diastolic filling, associated with rate and inadequate venous return (Figs. 73, 74, and 75).

THE NORMAL ST SEGMENT

After the QRS complex the phase of ventricular recovery begins. The early stage of recovery creates very small forces due to the size

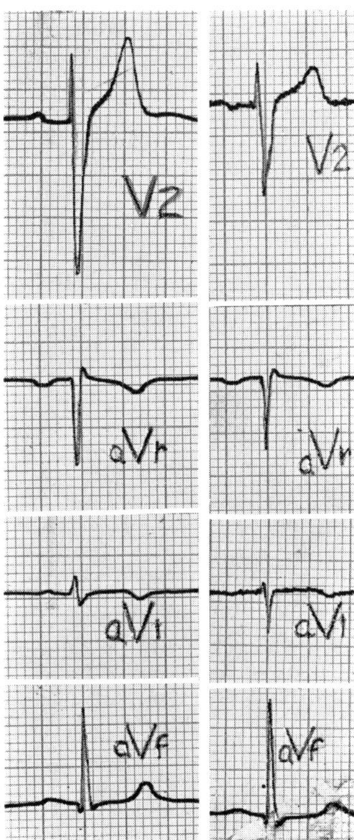

Figure 70. Note the small decrease in the terminal R wave in aVr from expiration (left) to inspiration (right).

and shape of the wave front. This early period is represented by a nearly isoelectric phase on the electrocardiogram and is called the ST segment. The initial anterior direction of the small forces originating from the right ventricle creates a normal elevation of the ST segment at V2. The proximity of the electrode at V2 position enhances this effect. Particularly in young individuals, normal ST segment elevations may be quite marked (Fig. 76). A slow cardiac rate is commonly associated with this finding. Normal ST segment elevation occurs in the leads with a positive wave for the entire event of ventricular recovery (leads with an upright T wave).

THE NORMAL T WAVE

Recovery of the left ventricle from apex to base creates a much larger force, manifested by the T wave. In general the T wave is positive in those leads with positive QRS complexes. Normal variations exist due to the difference in size, shape and speed in the wave front of recovery and excitation. The duration of the T wave reflects the time required for recovery. The main T wave deflection occupies roughly .16 sec. The entire recovery time from completion of QRS to completion of T approximates .28 to .36 sec. The T wave amplitude is greatest in the lead most nearly parallel to the greatest displacement of the T loop (allowing for electrode distance).

In the adult the T wave is normally upright in Leads I, II and precordial leads V3 through V6. Depending upon electrical axis and lead length the T wave may be either positive, negative or isoelectric in all other leads except aVr. Lead aVr normally has a negative T wave in the adult.

Amplitude of the T wave is very difficult to define in precise figures. In young individuals the T wave may be extraordinarily large. This is particularly true of the more athletic individual with a slow heart rate. In general a T wave of seven tenths millivolts (7 mm. at normal standard) is large, requiring consideration of age, rate, electrode distance and physiological stages.

The T wave is normally subject to variability. Drinking ice water to chill the apex reverses the apex base order of recovery inverting the T waves in those leads with positive electrodes facing the apex. Changes in cardiac filling due to change in cardiac rate, or changes in posture may also change the characteristic of the T wave.

The African ECG is particularly variable in reference to transitory T wave changes. A young adult negro with no demonstrable heart disease often presents a seeming abnormal record with a high degree of variability.* This is thought to

*Grusin, T.: Peculiarities of the African's Electrocardiogram and the Changes Observed in Serial Studies. *Circulation,* 9:866, 1954.

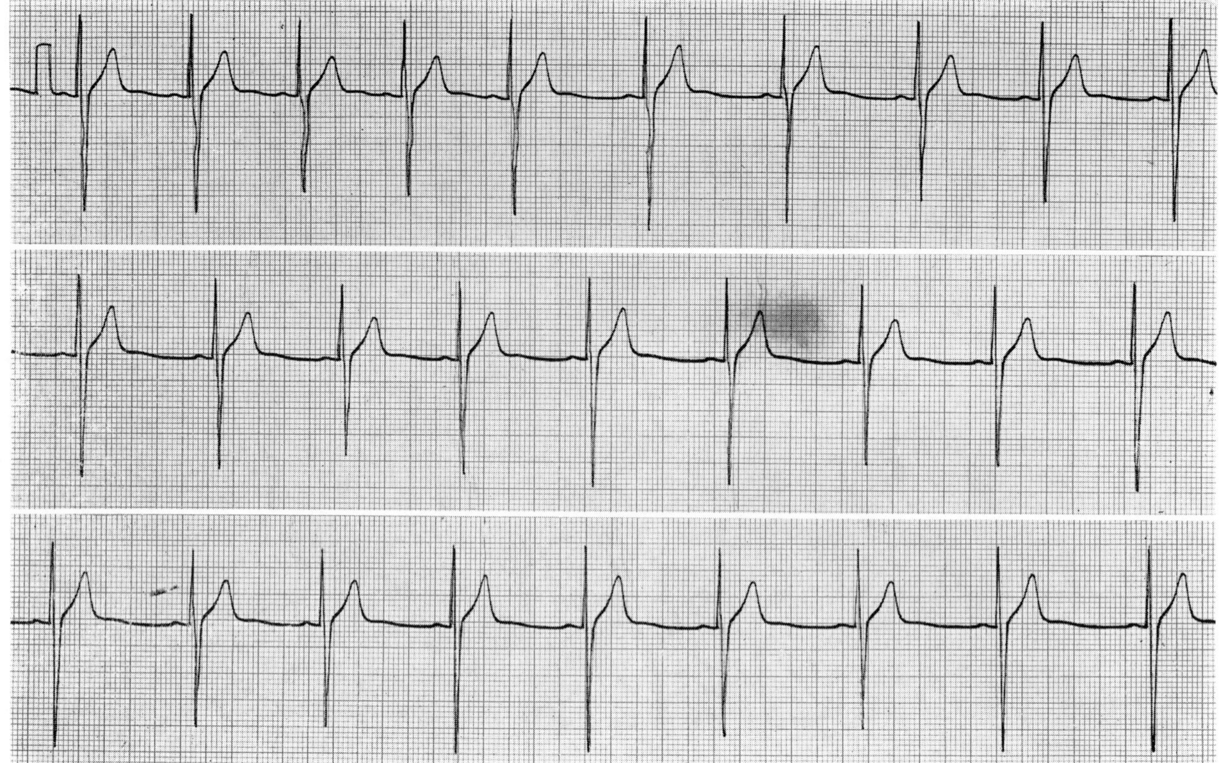

Figure 71. This is a continuous strip of Lead V2 showing the perfect Spirogram recorded by the S wave. Note there is no change in the R wave (first half of the QRS) and the base line is absolutely stable. This is a selective change of the S wave alone

occur more frequently during the time the juvenile pattern is changing to the adult characteristics (Fig. 77).

THE NORMAL U WAVE

The after potential force is demonstrated by a small positive wave immediately following the positive T wave. Little factual information regarding its normal and abnormal variations is available (Fig. 78).

THE NORMAL QT INTERVAL

The interval between the onset of ventricular excitation and the end of ventricular recovery is called the QT interval. This period of time corresponds approximately to mechanical systole of the heart, and is sometimes called electrical systole. The QT interval is properly measured as the longest interval in any of the leads. Its value will vary with the heart rate. The QT interval should be corrected for rate before determining whether it is within normal limits. This may be done by utilizing Bazette's formula:

$$K = \text{QT interval} \times \sqrt{\text{R} - \text{R interval}}$$

K is a constant and is .37 sec. for men and .40 sec. for women. R – R interval means the time between two successive R waves. The QT interval is measured directly from the tracing in question. Whenever QT interval times $\sqrt{R - R}$ is greater than the constant, K, the QT interval is prolonged. *An average QT interval is .34 to .44 sec.*

THE MEAN VECTOR

A number of normal values in electrocardiography are dependent upon the so called "mean vector." These are derived from the net positive or negative value of complexes graphed on the lead coordinates. The QRS complex, as an example, will have a net positive, negative or zero

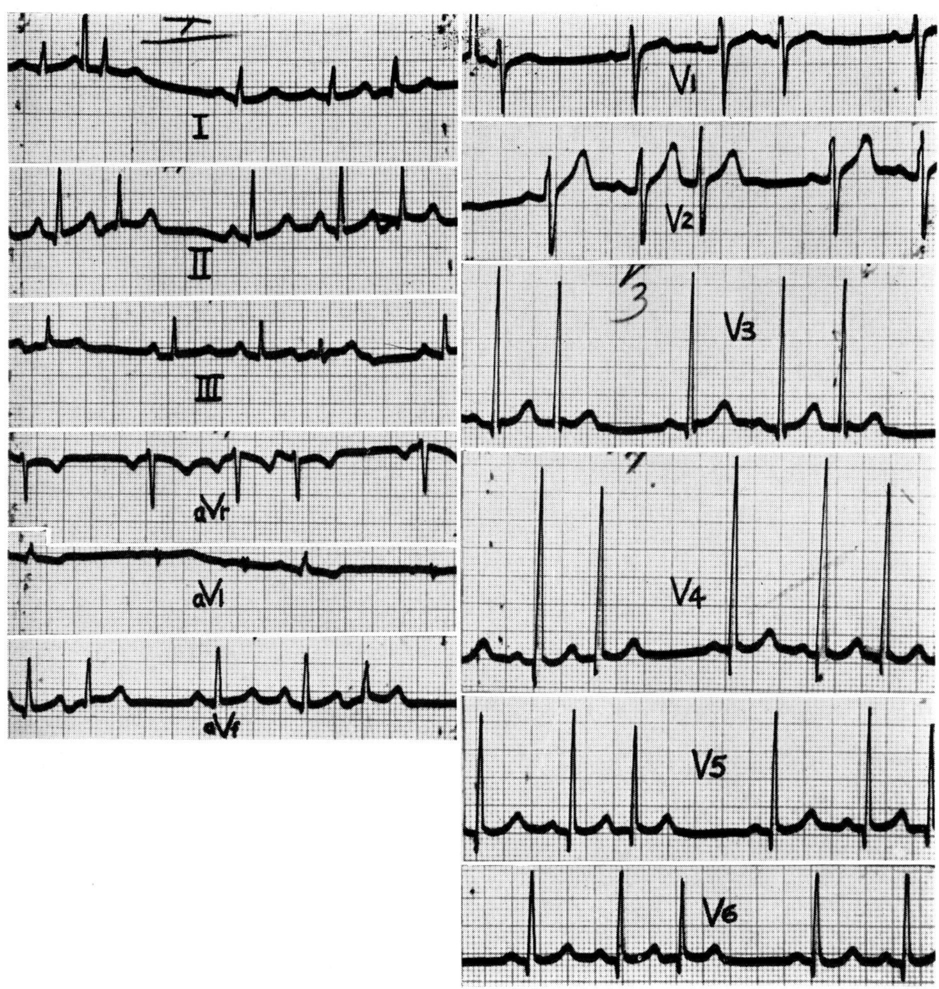

Figure 72. Each nodal premature contraction has less QRS amplitude than the preceding and following QRS complex. This appears to occur only with very early premature contractions.

value in any lead. The same is true for the other events. The final mean vector determined for an event is an over-all resultant force equated to the event.

The first step is to determine the net value of a complex in a given lead. The triangular area of the positive and negative deflection is obtained (amplitude times base divided by two). The values are subtracted (added algebraically) to obtain the net value. When the positive and negative deflections are equal the net value is zero. A lead with such a complex is called the isoelectrical lead for the event being measured. The mean vector is perpendicular to this lead. Given Lead I with a diphasic QRS complex and net value of zero, the mean QRS axis is perpendicular to Lead I. If Lead II and III are positive the mean QRS axis is +90°. Determination of the mean T and P vectors may be made in a similar manner.

The mean vector measurements are clearly mathematical derivatives and crude determinations. The reader should review again the mathematical origin of "mean" vectors obtained from coordinate graphs as discussed in Chapter I. They can be used for average directions and in a very coarse manner for magnitude.

THE MEAN .04 QRS VECTOR

On occasion it is advantageous to calculate the mean vector acting for a specific period of time. The mean QRS vector acting during the

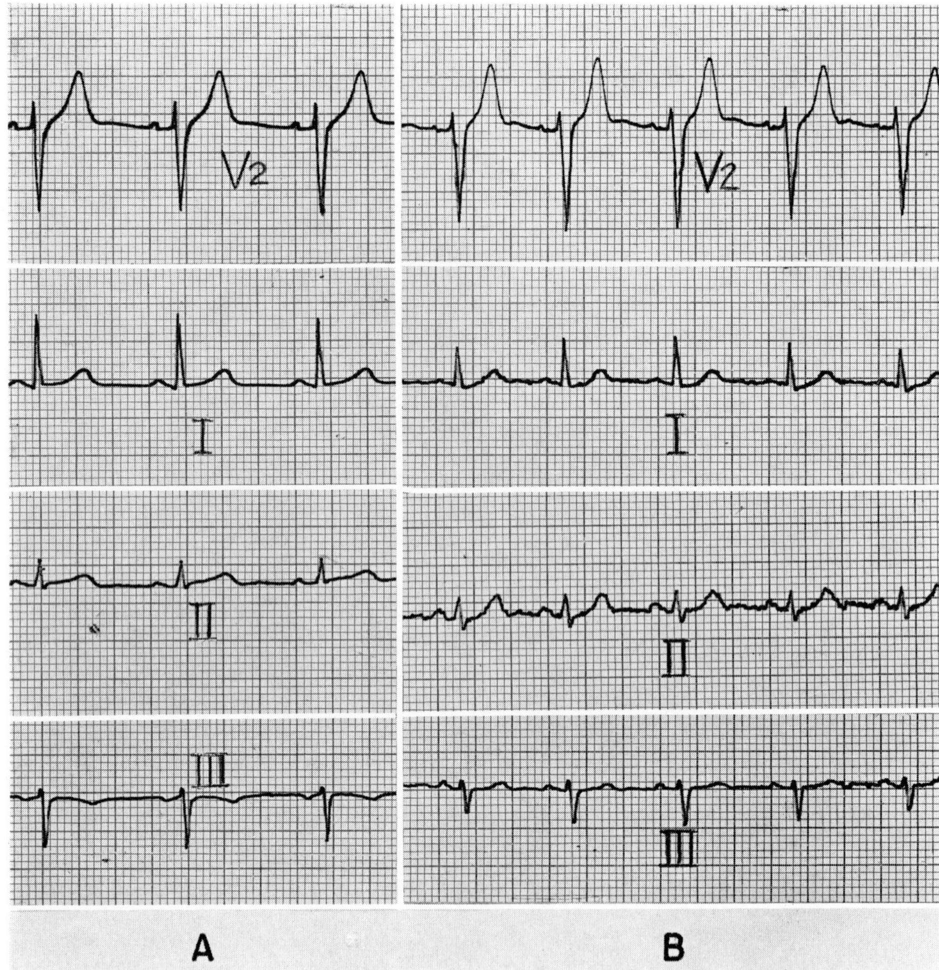

Figure 73. A) Before exercise, B) Immediately after exercise.

initial .04 sec. of ventricular excitation is manifested only during this .04 sec. interval, irrespective of the character of the QRS complex during the latter period of excitation. The terminal .04 sec. QRS vector acts only during the last .04 sec. of ventricular excitation.

The relationship of these component QRS vectors to the mean QRS vector may be illustrated by the following case (Fig. 79):

1) The total QRS duration is .08 sec. (longest QRS duration in any lead).

2) Lead III has a QRS duration of .08 sec. Its initial .04 sec. is a Q wave 4 mm. deep. The last .04 sec. is an R wave 4 mm. high. The initial .04 QRS value in minus 2 units (4 × 1 divided by 2), and its terminal QRS value is plus 2 (4 × 1 divided by 2). The mean QRS value in Lead III then, is 0.

3) Lead II has a QRS duration of only .04 sec. The complex has 8 mm. of positive amplitude. The mean QRS value in Lead II is 4 positive units (8 × 1 divided by 2). Since the QRS interval was short in Lead II, an isoelectric interval of .04 sec. duration must have occurred on this lead axis during ventricular excitation. This occurred either before or after the positive complex was inscribed.

4) Lead I has a QRS duration of .08 sec. The entire complex is positive. Its height of 4 mm. is reached at .04 sec. The initial .04 sec. QRS value is plus 2 units (4 × 1 divided by 2). The terminal .04 QRS value is also plus 2 units. The mean QRS value in Lead I is plus 4 units (4 × 2 divided by 2).

The initial .04 QRS value changes from minus 2 units in Lead III, to plus 2 units in Lead I.

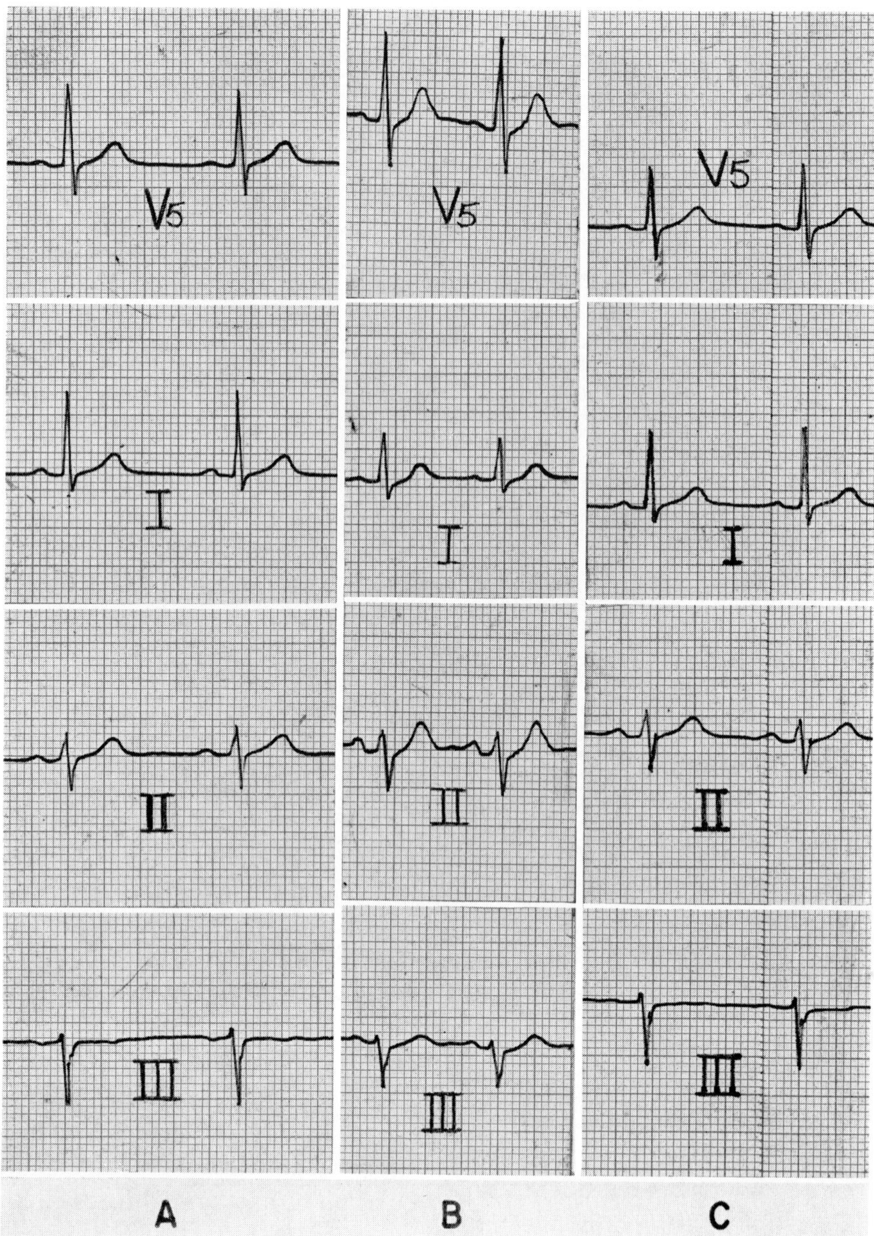

Figure 74. A) Before exercise, B) Immediately after exercise, C) Return to normal rate after exercise.

Therefore, an isoelectric point must exist between Lead I and Lead III for the initial .04 vector. This isoelectric point was at Lead II and wrote an isoelectric interval before the positive wave occurred. This also caused the QRS interval to appear shortened in Lead II (.04 sec.). The initial .04 mean QRS vector is perpendicular to the lead axis of Lead II and directed toward Lead I, or its axis is –30°. The terminal .04 mean QRS vector records plus 2 units in Lead III, plus 2 units in Lead I and plus 4 units in Lead II. Its axis is parallel to the axis of Lead II or +60°. The mean QRS complex is perpendicular to Lead III where the mean QRS magnitude was 0. The mean QRS vector has an axis of +30°.

The anterior or posterior direction of the .04 sec. vector can be determined from the V leads, again by locating the transition from positive to negative value.

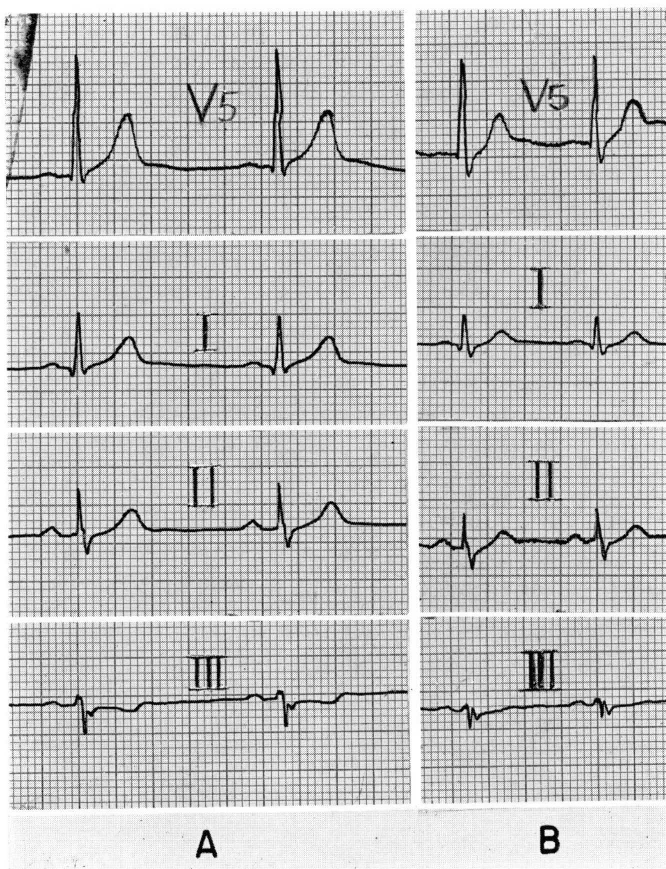

Figure 75. A) Before exercise, B) Immediately after exercise.

NORMAL MEAN QRS AXIS

The projection of the QRS vector on the frontal plane is called the QRS axis. It is defined in degrees from the axis of Lead I. The normal adult heart may have a QRS axis between –30° and +110°. Any axis beyond this range must be explained before the axis is considered normal. In the infant the axis is normally to the right, beyond +90°, and gradually shifts leftward to assume the adult position. As age advances, the QRS axis commonly shifts leftward to an axis of 0° or a minus value.

As the QRS vector is rotated out of the frontal plane to either a more posterior or anterior direction, its magnitude in the frontal plane is diminished. In the normal adult the mean QRS vector is directed posteriorly. This is the influence of early completion of septal activation, causing the terminal QRS pathway to be directed posteriorly. If the left ventricle is elongated the septal content is larger and the mean QRS vector is directed even more leftward and backward.

The axis of the QRS vector in the frontal plane, or any other plane, can be determined by the methods outlined previously for the calculation of any spatial force in any plane.

THE MEAN T VECTOR

The spatial T vector is directed far to the right and posteriorly at birth. The vector gradually moves leftward and anteriorly with age. Occasionally the posterior direction of the T vector may persist into adult life. This is one cause of negative T waves in V1 through V3 and it is called a persistent juvenile pattern.

The normal mean T vector in the adult approximates the longitudinal axis of the left ven-

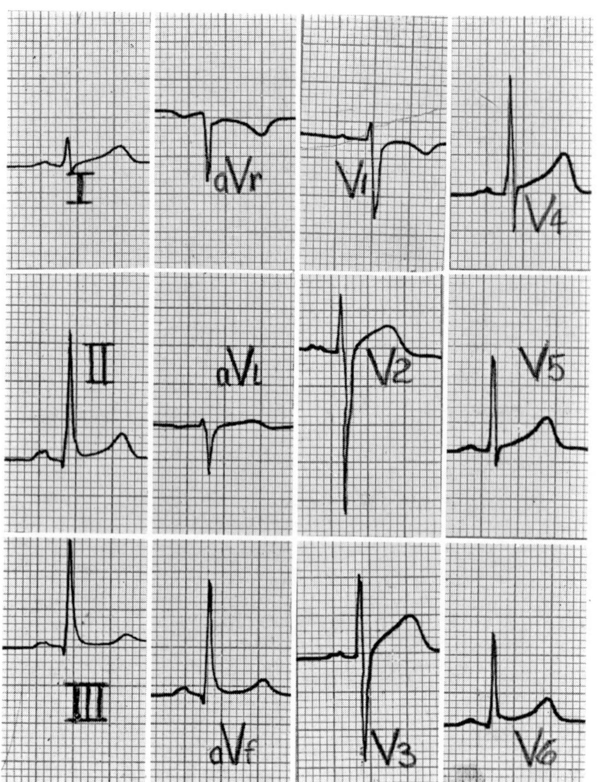

Figure 76. Note ST segment elevation in Leads II, III, aVf, V2 and V3 in a healthy subject.

tricle. Thus it is normally anterior to the mean QRS vector. When the mean QRS vector becomes markedly leftward the mean T vector will be to its right, e.g., QRS –30°, T vector zero degrees.

The magnitude of the normal T vector is usually less than the magnitude of the QRS vector, although it may be larger in slow hearts with vertical axis as seen in young individuals.

THE MEAN SPATIAL QRS-T ANGLE

Chiefly due to early completion of septal activation a normal angle exists between the mean QRS and mean T vectors (Fig. 80). The spatial angle in the adult is usually less than 60°. Occasional individuals without known evidence of heart disease may have an angle as large as 90°. These are exceptional. Any angle over 60° must be explained.

In the normal young adult the ventricules are short. The septal component is small. The mean QRS vector tends to be electrically vertical and not very far posterior. It is chiefly straight down. The QRS and T vectors are nearly parallel and the mean spatial, QRS-T angle may be only 15°. Later in life the left ventricle tends to elongate, increasing the ef-

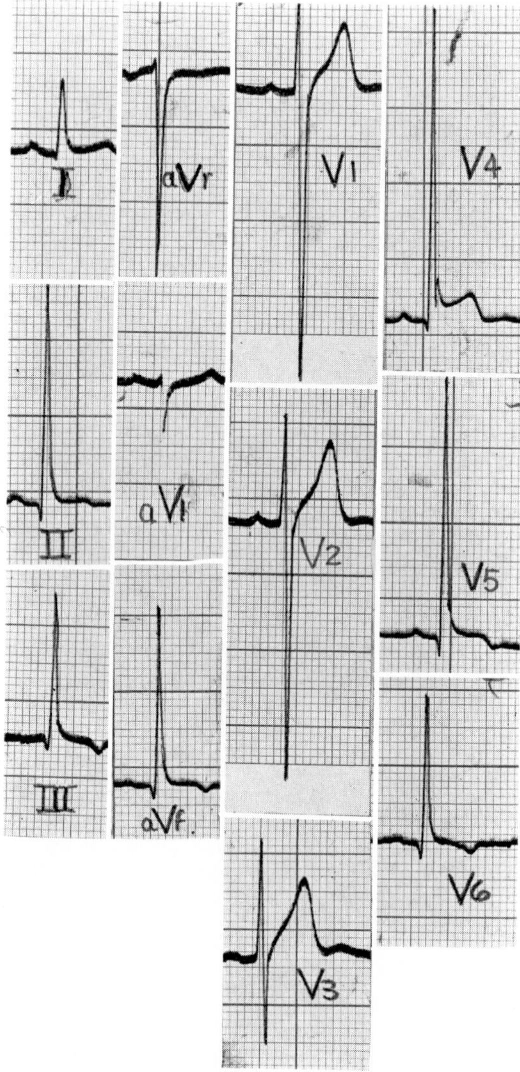

Figure 77. This ECG was recorded on a young negro without any demonstrable evidence of heart disease, hypertrophy or hypertension. The QRS amplitude is increased, in part, due to the small chest. Note the QRS complex being recorded off the paper. This is an error in technique. When the QRS amplitude is too large for proper recording, the standardization should be reduced.

fective magnitude of the septal arc vector. This causes a shift in mean QRS axis leftward and posterior. The mean spatial QRS-T angle widens.

If the magnitude, direction and sense of the QRS and T vector is known, the net positive or negative value that is recorded in any lead can be determined (Fig. 80).

If the spatial QRS-T angle is abnormally wide, it will register abnormal patterns measured by individual leads. The measurement of the QRS-T angle projection on only one plane is fallacious and misleading. In any instance when the QRS and T vector have the same frontal plane axis, the mean QRS-T angle in the frontal plane is 0°. If the QRS vector is posterior and the T vector is anterior, the spatial angle will become smaller as it becomes vertical

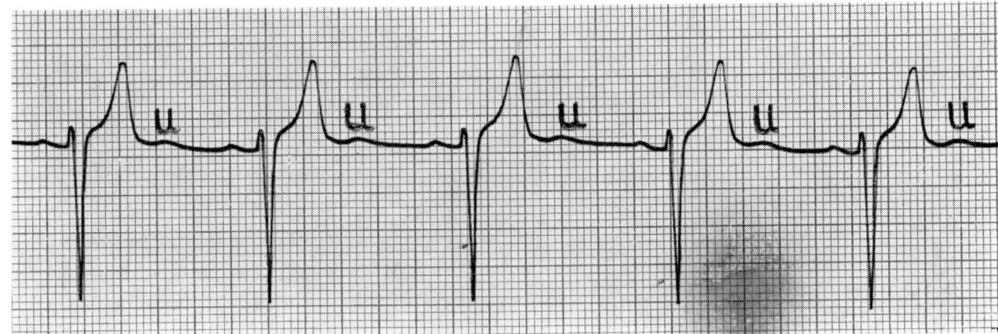

Fiigure 78.

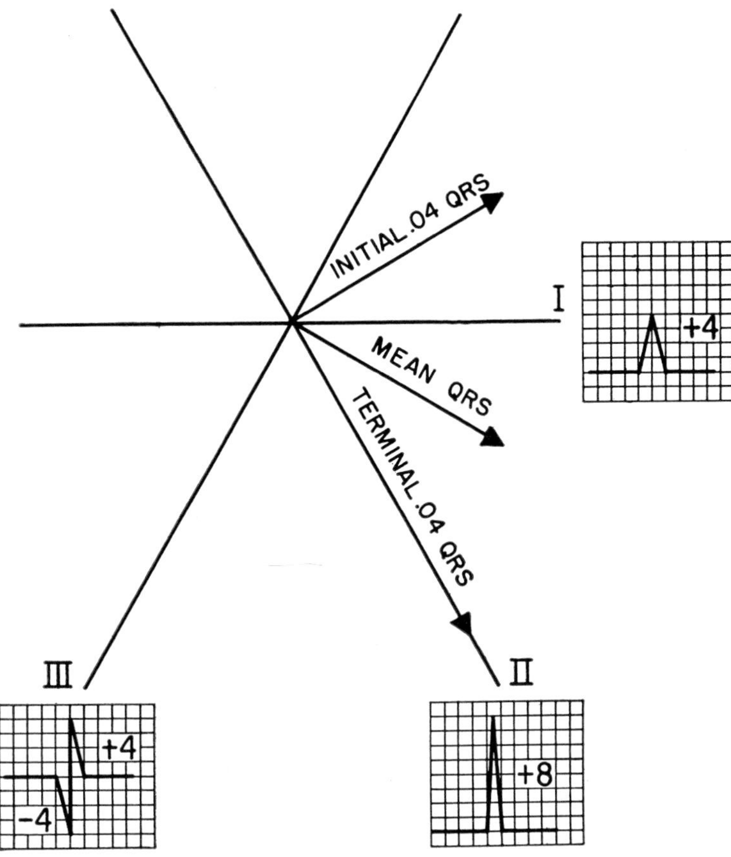

Figure 79.

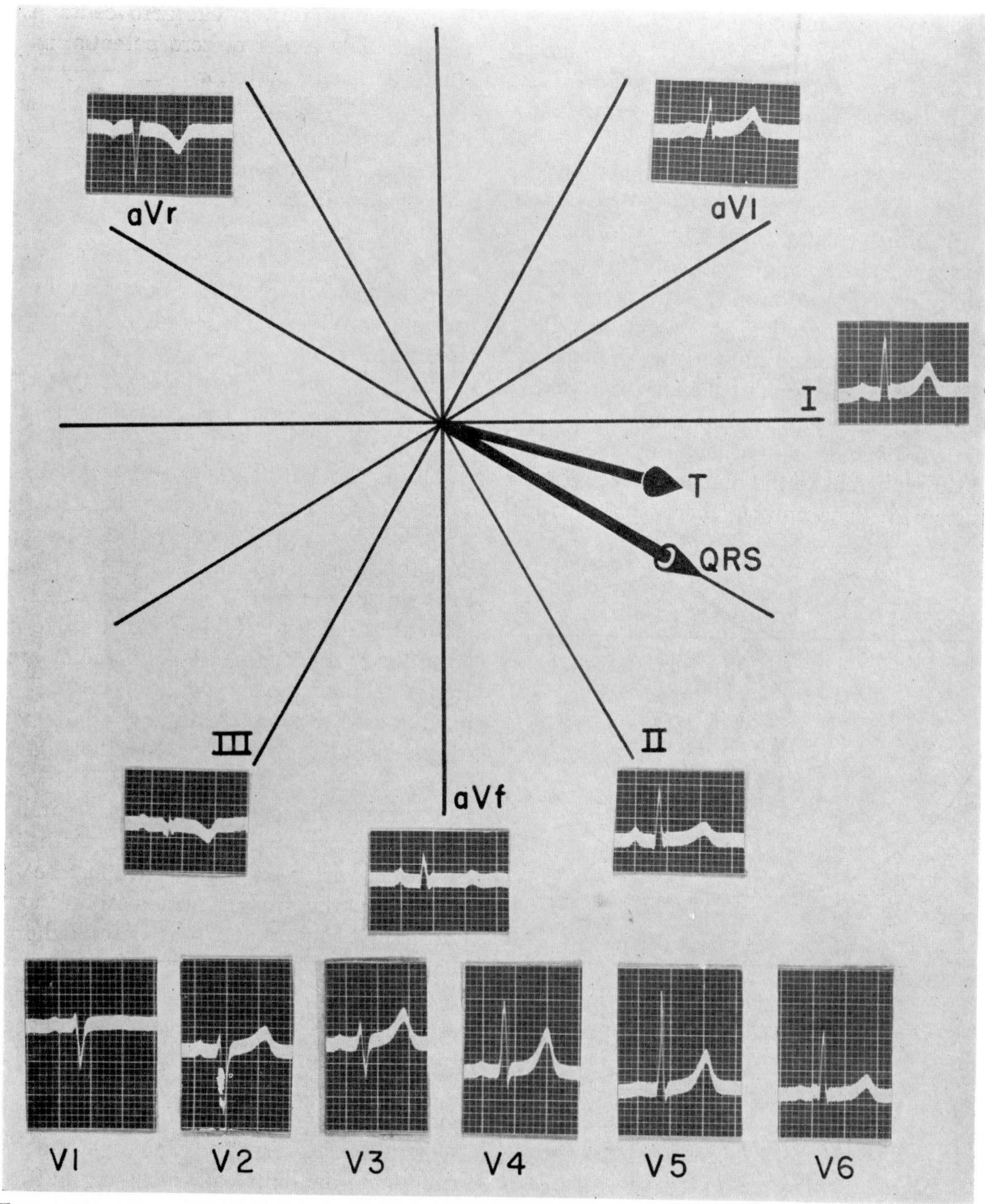

Figure 80. Mean QRS axis +30°, with transition at V3; mean T axis +15°, with transition at V1. The mean spatial QRS-T angle is 40°.

(Fig. 81). Viewed in the sagittal plane, the angle between a and b is larger than the more vertical angle between a′ and b′, although in both cases the angle is 0 as projected on the frontal plane, and 60° as projected on the transverse plane.

If the QRS and T vectors both have an axis of +90°, the angle will be either 0 or 180° in the transverse plane projection. Further increase in the spatial angle will only increase the magnitude of projection in the transverse plane (Fig. 81). This accounts for the wide QRS-T angle in the V leads in the presence of a vertical electrical axis and small mean spatial QRS-T angle.

Certain difficulties in calculating the spatial angle are inherent to the human body and must be assumed. Not only is there an individual anatomic variation in the V lead position, but the location of the cardiac zero center is not constant. The center of zero potential may be either anterior or posterior to its expected location, or it may be lower or higher. When the zero center is shifted, the entire reference system is altered. Nevertheless, it is better to have some means of approximating the spatial angle than none at all.

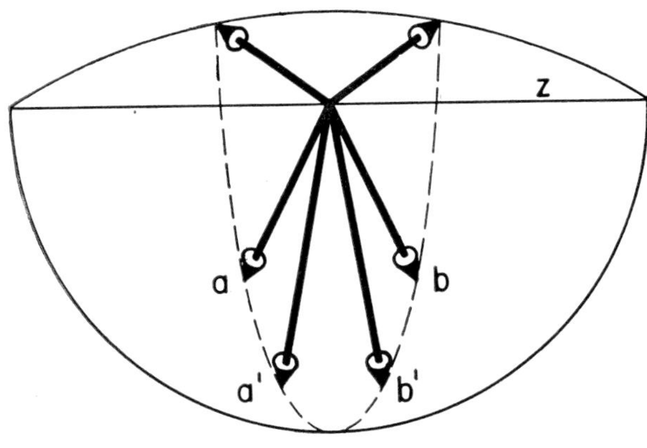

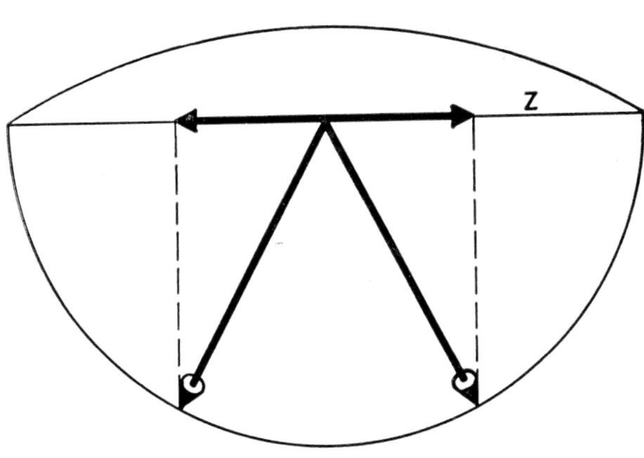

Figure 81.

The actual calculation of the spatial QRS-T angle is somewhat cumbersome and for this reason a simplified table is provided to approximate readily the spatial QRS-T angle (see spatial angle chart). Each vector is described by its axis in the frontal plane and its transition point in the V leads. The description of the vector in the left-hand margin is located for either the QRS or T vector. The description of the other vector is located at the bottom of the table. At the intersection of the columns, the value of the spatial angle is recorded. The method of using the table is exactly like using an ordinary mileage chart. The values are accurate mathematically within 5°. The chart may be used to calculate any two spatial vector forces including the angle between .04 QRS vectors and the mean QRS vector.

Assuming the lead axis of V6 is parallel to the X coordinate, when a complex is transitional at V6 the vector for that event must be +90° or –90° in the frontal plane. Accordingly, a transition complex at V6 is described in the chart as a strictly vertical force of +90° or –90°. If the vector is only slightly posterior, V1 through V5 will be negative. If it is slightly anterior, V6 is negative. The more anterior or posterior the direction of the spatial force, the smaller its magnitude in Lead aVf.

Transition at V6 with a diphasic or isoelectric value in all the limb leads including aVf is produced by a vector which is directed entirely anteriorly or posteriorly. Such a vector is truly perpendicular to the frontal plane. If it is anterior, V1 through V5 are positive. If the vector is directed posteriorly V1 through V5 are negative. On the chart they are described as anterior to the frontal plane with transition at V6

(A, V6) or posterior to the frontal plane with transition at V6 (P, V6).

In any individual case the spatial angle between two forces can be determined by using the law of cosines (Fig. 82). If a line is drawn between the terminations of the QRS and T vectors, a spatial triangle is formed. By the law

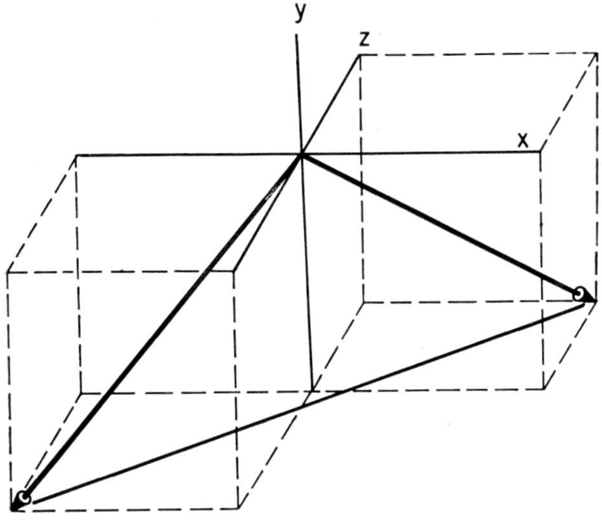

Figure 82.

of cosines the angles of any triangle can be determined whenever the magnitudes of the three sides are known. One side of the triangle is the QRS vector and another side is the T vector. The base (B) must be calculated. The base can be calculated because the twelve lead ECG measures the spatial force along three perpendicular axes; X, Y, and Z. The projection of the force on each axis is known for both the QRS and T vector. The sum of the square of difference of projected magnitude in each coordinate equals the square of the base. This may be expressed:

$$(X_{qrs} - X_t)^2 + (Y_{qrs} - Y_t)^2 + (Z_{qrs} - Z_t)^2 = B^2.$$

Utilizing the law of cosines the

$$\text{cosine of the QRS-T Angle} = \frac{(\text{QRS vector})^2 + (\text{T vector})^2 - B^2}{2 \times \text{QRS vector} \times \text{T vector}}$$

Stepwise one determines,

1) The spatial magnitude of the QRS vector
2) the spatial magnitude of the T vector
3) the value of Base squared
4) and the cosine of the QRS-T Angle by the law of cosines.

VIII

Fundamentals of Vectorcardiography

THE PREVIOUS DISCUSSIONS have emphasized that the electrical events of the heart describe spatial pathways or loops, P, QRS, and T. The vectorcardiogram strives to record these spatial loops. The spatial loops are polygons, and the ECG records the successive resultants of the polygon. The differences and similarities of the VCG and ECG are those which exist between polygons and coordinate graphs of polygon resultants. It is clear that the ECG measures duration, sequence and direction. The VCG also measures magnitude because it records the sides of the polygon as the spatial pathway.

The Frontal Plane. Vectorcardiograms are recorded with a cathode ray oscilloscope. Use is made of the X and Y axis of the cathode ray beam (side to side and up and down) created by the horizontal and vertical plates. The lead chosen to represent the X coordinate is fed into the X axis. The lead representing the Y coordinate is fed into the Y axis. When the X and Y coordinates are recorded simultaneously they record the frontal plane projection of spatial loops (Fig. 83). The six limb leads of the ECG can be extracted from this projection.

The Sagittal Plane projection of the spatial loops requires use of the Z and Y coordinate leads. The lead representing the Z coordinate is fed into the X axis of the oscilloscope. The Y coordinate lead is fed into the Y axis. Their simultaneous recording is the sagittal plane of the spatial loops (Fig. 84).

When an oscilloscope with two beams is used, the sagittal and frontal plane projections of the vectorcardiogram can be recorded simultaneously. This gives a frontal and profile view of any one cardiac cycle. The two planes utilize all three mutually perpendicular coordinates (X, Y, Z) thus defining spatial forces.

The Transverse Plane is recorded by feeding the lead for X coordinate into the X axis and

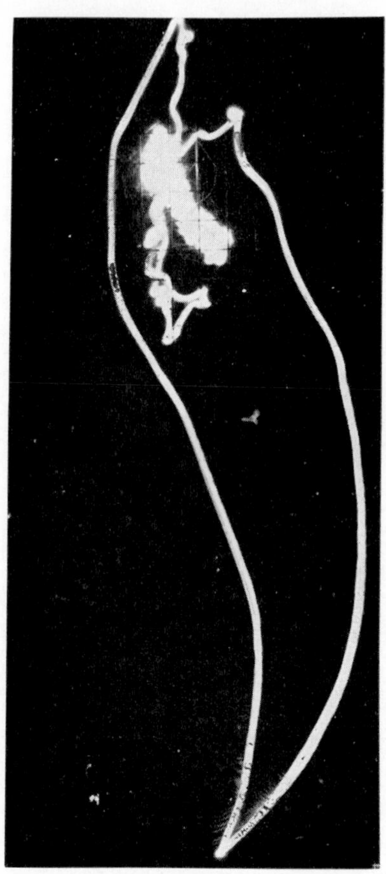

Figure 83.

the lead for the Z coordinate into the Y axis (Fig. 85). The transverse plane represents the cross section through the thorax. The V leads may be extracted from the transverse plane by

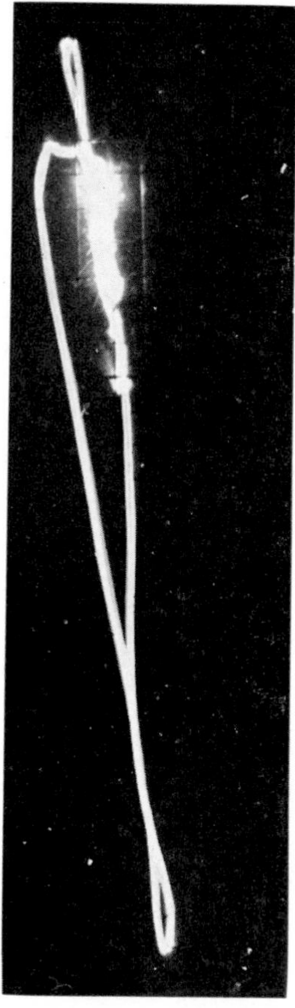

Figure 84.

projecting the transverse plane upon the coordinate axis of each V lead.

Timing is accomplished by introducing interruptions in the beam at known intervals (Fig. 86). If the beam is blanked out each .0025 sec. an interruption will occur in the loop every .0025 sec. By locating the time intervals on both the frontal and sagittal planes the point in space for each instantaneous vector can be described in terms of its X, Y, Z coordinates. From such a determination a spatial representation of the spatial pathway (polygon) can be constructed. The instantaneous vectors of such a three dimensional representation are the successive resultants of the sides of the polygon. The successive instantaneous spatial vectors can be projected upon each lead axis to construct each lead (Fig. 87).

It is obvious that whatever leads one uses for X, Y, Z coordinates can in turn be extracted from their recorded vectorcardiogram. This in no way validates these particular leads as true representatives of X, Y, Z coordinates for the body. In any system employing bipolar leads, the leads must be centered in reference to the zero center and the leads standardized equally to each other. Standardization requires that both the lead length and the radius distance of the electrodes from the zero center be known.

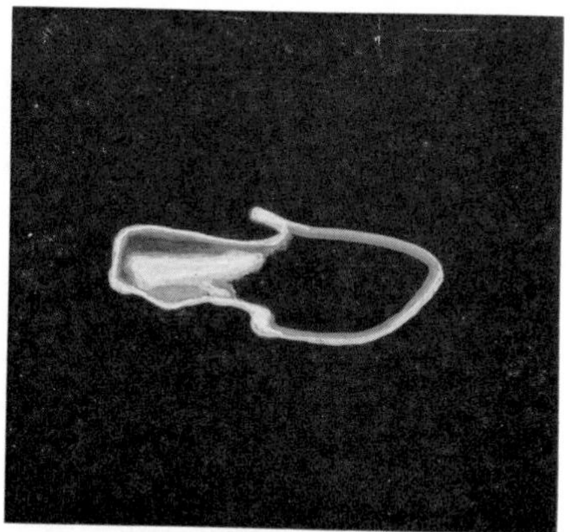

Figure 85.

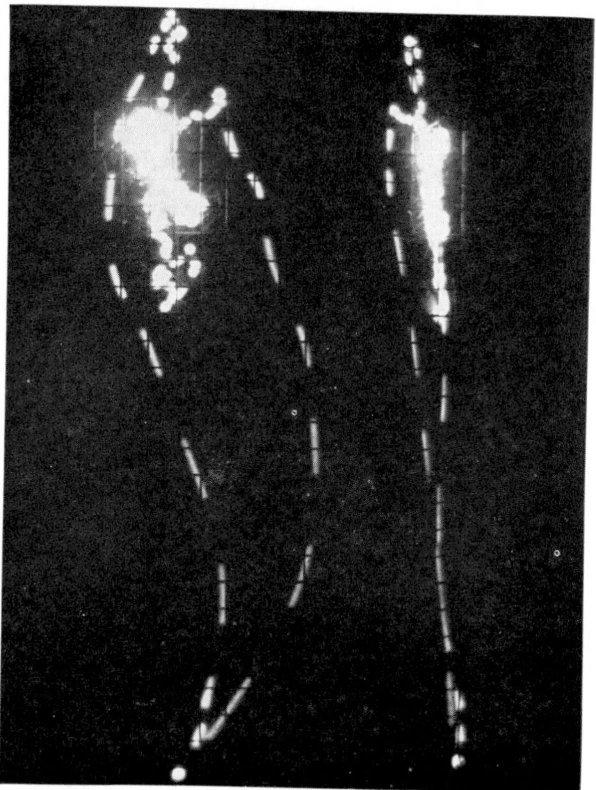

Figure 86.

THE VCG SYSTEM

The system used to record the vectorcardiograms demonstrated in this text attempts to satisfy the requirements of: 1) symmetrical relation to the zero center, 2) measured lead lengths, and 3) known radius distances of electrodes from the zero center. The first step is location of the zero center. It is assumed that the center of the left ventricle approximates this point. A left lateral and PA chest X-ray is obtained. In each subject the center is located as: a) one half the vertical distance between the right atrial groove and the left leaf of the diaphragm, b) one half the distance between the mid sternal line and the left cardiac border at this level, and c) one half the distance between the anterior and posterior cardiac borders at the same vertical level as located on the sagittal X-ray (Fig. 88).

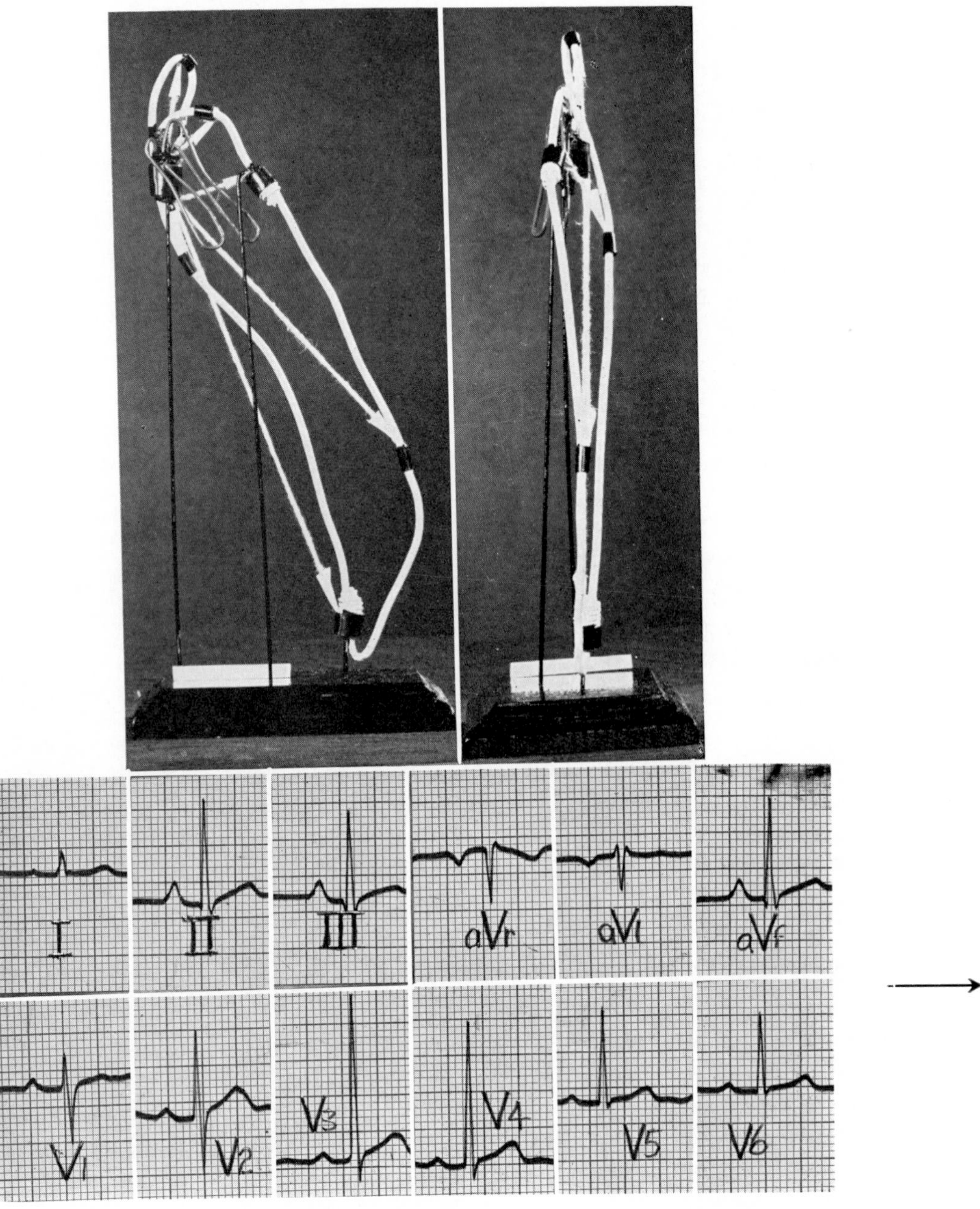

The transverse lead (X coordinate) is on the back across the shoulders. It is arranged so that its length is bisected by a perpendicular extending to the cardiac center previously measured. In the adult the length most often chosen is 22 cm. Thus if the center is 4 cm. to the left of the mid spinal line the left electrode (+) is 15 cm. to the left of the midline and the right electrode (−) 7 cm. to the right of the midline. The narrowness of the lower part of the thorax prevents symmetrical location of a lead of such length at this location in most normal adults. For this reason the lead is placed across the upper thorax. It is desirable to retain lead length whenever possible.*

The vertical lead (Y coordinate) is bisected by a perpendicular from it to the cardiac center. The usual lead length in the adult is 30 cm. The negative electrode is the same as the right electrode for the transverse lead. The positive electrode is directly 30 cm. beneath it.

The three symmetrically placed electrodes are all of equal radius distance from the center. The chief difference in their sensitivity is their difference in lead length. Since the vertical lead is the longest it will have the greatest sensitivity.

*It is recognized that the left shoulder has a more complicated potential field. However, the advantages gained by a long lead length symmetrical to the zero center outweigh this disadvantage.

In order that they be equal the standardization (amplification) must be adjusted. This is done simply by multiplying the transverse lead standardization by the ratio of the lead lengths. With a standardization of 1.0 cm. = 1 mv. for the transverse lead (length 22 cm.), the vertical lead (30 cm.) standardization should be .73 cm. = 1 mv.

$$1.00 \times \frac{22}{30} = .73.$$

The sagittal lead (Z coordinate) is a V lead placed directly over the cardiac center on the back (commonly 4 cm. to the left of the mid spine). The standard Wilson central terminal is utilized. The lead length is obtained by measuring the distance on the sagittal X-ray from the center to the back (commonly 19 cm.). The standardization is determined by using the equation for the sensitivity of the bipolar lead ($3L/R^3$) and the V lead ($3/r^2$). When the standardization for the transverse lead is 1.0 cm. = 1 mv. (transverse lead 22 cm. long, vertical lead 30 cm. long and sagittal lead 19 cm. long) the formula is:

$$\text{V lead standardization} = \frac{r^2 \times \text{transverse lead length;}}{R^3}$$

$$.42 = \frac{19 \times 19 \times 22}{18800}$$

Like all systems, leading from the human body, certain errors must be assumed. The indi-

Figure 87. The three dimensional VCG model is constructed from a simultaneously recorded frontal and sagittal plane VCG (frontal view at the left and sagittal view at the right). The very large white loop is the QRS loop. The black markers represent .01 sec. intervals. The white vectors are the instantaneous spatial vectors at each .01 sec. (the resultants of the polygon). The QRS loop begins anteriorly and sweeps downward, to the left and posterior. Its terminal portion is complicated reflecting the terminal complications of the wave front. The sagittal presentation is a left profile of the model. The small P loop in this instance is more vertical than the more leftward T loop.

The white marker at the base of the model represents 5 cm. length and is a standardization. By comparing the site of the standard in each succeeding photograph, a concept of relative size can be appreciated. All succeeding models, unless otherwise stated, are built to the same scale, in terms of electrical moment (corrected for lead length and distance of electrode positions from the heart). Each centimeter equals 9.5 millivolts as electrical moment.

The above example depicts a vertical QRS loop. Note the initial Q wave in Lead III corresponding to the initial upward course of the QRS loop and the terminal S wave in Lead II, Lead III, and aVf as the terminal QRS pathway is directed even farther toward the right shoulder. This event also creates a terminal R wave in aVr and aVl. As the terminal QRS pathway is nearly perpendicular to the axis of Lead I, it has almost no influence on that lead.

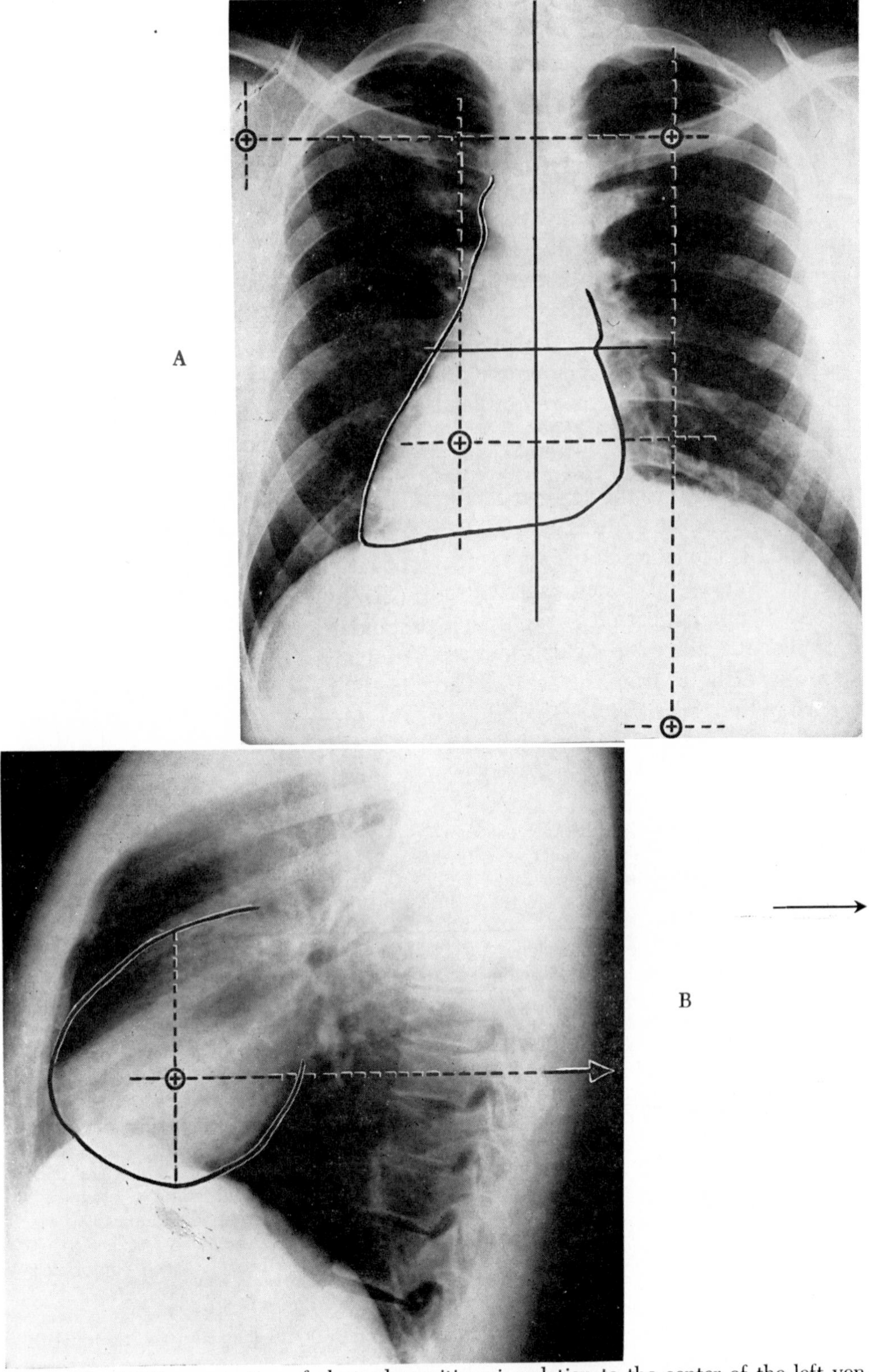

Figure 88. A) Demonstration of electrode positions in relation to the center of the left ventricle as seen on the PA film. B) Demonstration of the method of determining the sagittal lead length from the sagittal x-ray. C) Diagram of actual electrode placement for recording VCGs.

vidual variation in body shape, body size, and the location of the zero center are in part corrected in this system. It also enables conversion for factors of radius distance and lead length from one subject to the next (terms of electrical moment) which cannot be done unless such measurements are made. Without such conversion factors electrocardiographic and vectorcardiographic measurements of magnitude are invalid. Unless the leads are standardized in relation to each other, the loops are distorted.

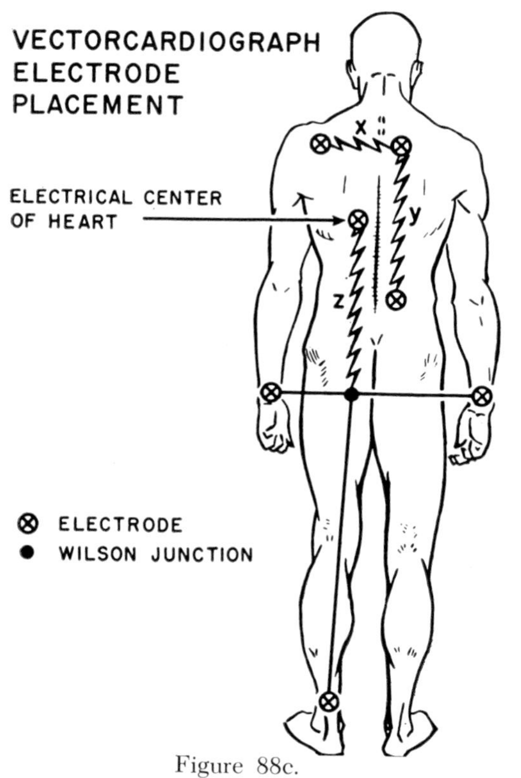

Figure 88c.

The general configuration of the complexes of P, QRS, T in the 12 lead routine ECG leads can be extracted from the VCG. Simply draw the lead axis through the center of the vectorcardiogram and graph the instantaneous vectors on the lead axis like a simple coordinate graph. Differences between the extracted leads and recorded leads can be attributed to difference in the lead systems employed. The routine ECG makes no corrections for zero center location, lead lengths or radius distance.

INDEX OF MAXIMUM POTENTIAL AND POTENTIAL SECONDS

The vectorcardiogram enables the calculation of the *Index of Maximum Potential* and the *Index of Potential Seconds.* The former is directly related to left ventricular surface area (and consequently stroke volume) and the latter is an expression of wall thickness as well. The index of maximum potential is obtained for the left ventricle simply by measuring the length of the QRS pathway after completion of right ventricular and septal activation. The pathway represents the length of the sides of the polygon.

The instantaneous long left ventricular vector commonly represents the resultant of the base vector and septal vector. Thus the last half of the QRS has two major directions: 1) a longitudinal and 2) a posterior component. The longitudinal component represents the area of the base and the posterior component represents the area of the septum. These two components are roughly two sides of a triangle (semiparallelogram) and the long left ventricle vector is the diagonal or their resultant.

The index of potential seconds is obtained by first multiplying the length of each segment of the spatial pathway by its duration of action then summing these values. Each segment represents a side of the polygon or a component force expressed in millivolts thus each segment is converted to millivolts times sec./100.

Since the difference in time of onset for endocardial excitation for different muscle regions is not great, it is practical to begin at .00 sec. for the onset of action for a force. Thus the side of the polygon from .04 sec. to .05 sec. has an average duration of .045 sec. The length of the side depicts the magnitude of the force, e.g., 3 mv. In such a case 3 mv. × .045 sec. = 13.5 × sec./100.

This value represents the force in units of time manifested by this one side of the polygon. A similar procedure should be done for each successive side. The sum expressed in mv. × sec./100 is an index of the voltage in units of time created by the left ventricle for one cardiac cycle.

In order to be comparable from one subject to the next the index of maximum potential and the index of potential seconds must be converted to terms of electrical moment by multiplying by the factor $R^3/3L$. This factor is the reciprocal of the sensitivity the transverse lead used as a base for standardization. The index of maximum potential and index of potential seconds are determined per cardiac cycle, to be expressed per minute they must be multiplied by the pulse rate (Fig. 89).

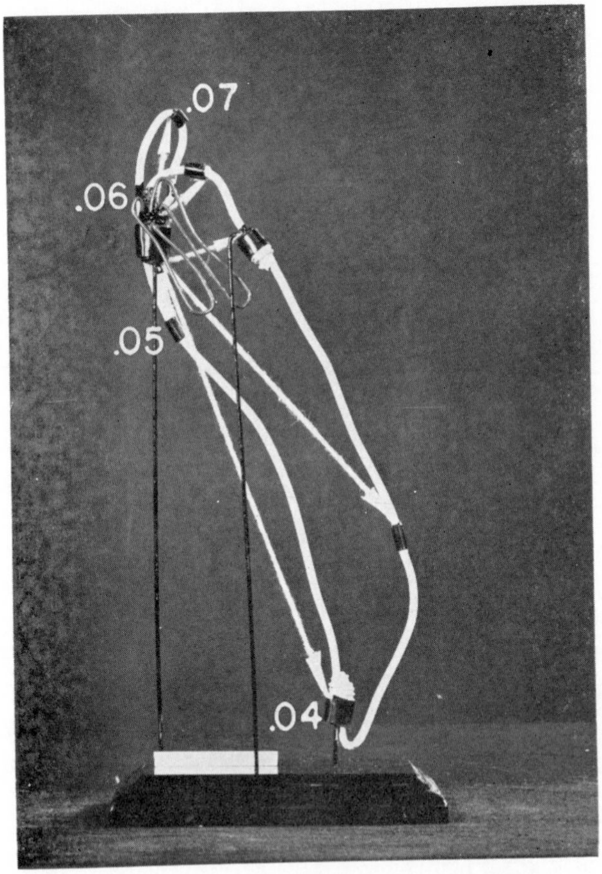

Figure 89. In the above example the QRS duration is .09 sec. (the .08 time marker is behind the T loop). The long left ventricular vector occurs at .04 sec. The length of the pathway from .04 to .09 sec. is the index of maximum potential. In this case the length is 31.5 cm. or 299.25 mv. (1 cm. equals 9.5 mv. in terms of electrical moment). The lengths for each time interval for calculation of potential seconds are as follows:

.04 – .05 sec. =	16 cm. =	152 mv. =	684 mv. sec./100
.05 – .06 sec. =	6 cm. =	57 mv. =	313.5 mv. sec./100
.06 – .07 sec. =	4.5 cm. =	42.8 mv. =	278.2 mv. sec./100
.07 – .08 sec. =	4 cm. =	38 mv. =	305.0 mv. sec./100
.08 – .09 sec. =	1 cm. =	9.5 mv. =	80.8 mv. sec./100
			1661.5 mv. sec./100

or 1.66 volts × sec./100 equals the potential seconds per QRS cycle. At a cardiac rate of 80 per minute the potential seconds per minutes would be 1.66 volts × sec./100 × 80 or 132.8 volts × sec./100 or 1.33 volt sec. per minute.

THE NORMAL VECTORCARDIOGRAM

The normal vectorcardiogram depicts a QRS loop to the right at birth. It is of small magnitude in terms of electrical moment (Fig. 90). There is a gradual transition to the adult type vectorcardiogram. In the child the values obtained from the VCG (index of maximum potential and index of potential seconds) remains small (Fig. 91). The values increase with increasing body size until early adult life. From this peak there appears to be a decline in the size of the VCG. The average forty year old American male has a decrease in index of maximum potential. The significance of this is not clear. Theoretically it could represent changes in density of charge across the wave front secondarily related to cell function, or even a decrease in cardiac output. Common types of normal vectorcardiograms are illustrated for the reader to compare with the routine ECG (Figs. 92, 93, 94, and 95).

The VCG in athletic individuals is usually much larger with a large index of maximum potential and a large index of potential seconds, per cardiac cycle. These individuals commonly have slow pulse rates with large stroke volumes. The surface area of the ventricles is greater, increasing the size of the excitation wave front manifested by an increased index of maximum potential. The ST interval is often displaced and the T loops are increased in magnitude. The increase in T magnitude is evidence of physiological enlargement rather than pathological change.

Characteristically, the QRS loop of the athlete is opened, consistent with cardiac dilatation. The terminal portion of the loop is often complicated indicating a complicated wave front at the base of the dilated ventricle (Figs. 96 and 97).

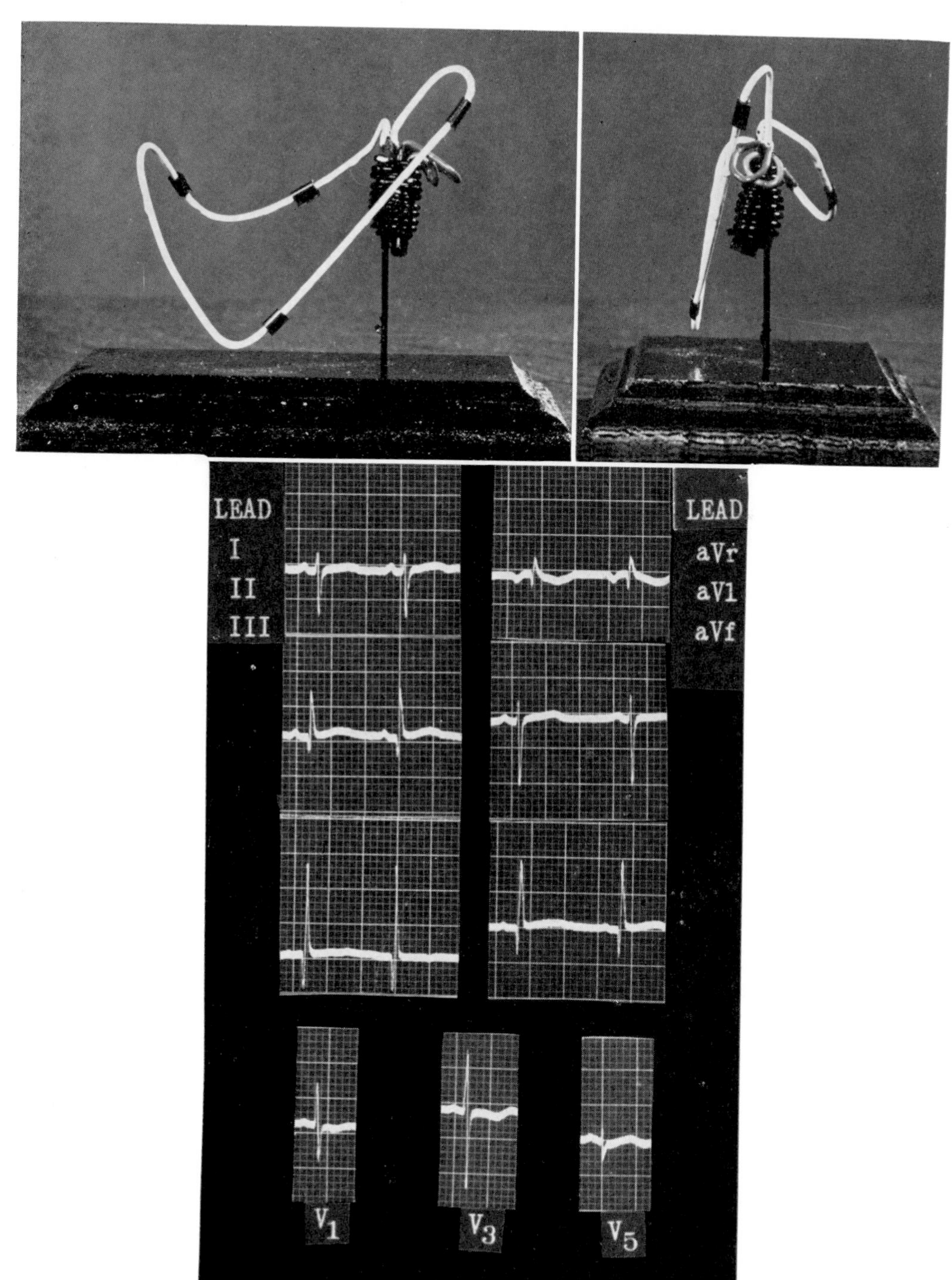

Figure 90. A vectorcardiogram of a seven day old infant. Note the rightward direction of the QRS loop and the mean QRS axis on the ECG of + 120°. The initial R wave in Lead I is depicted by the initial leftward course of the QRS loop. The terminal S wave depicts the rightward course of the loop. Try to reconstruct the character of the QRS complex in each of the other six limb leads by projecting the loop on the correct lead axis. The QRS duration is only .05 sec. This model is the only one not corrected for electrical moment as it was recorded by a different technique in 1951.

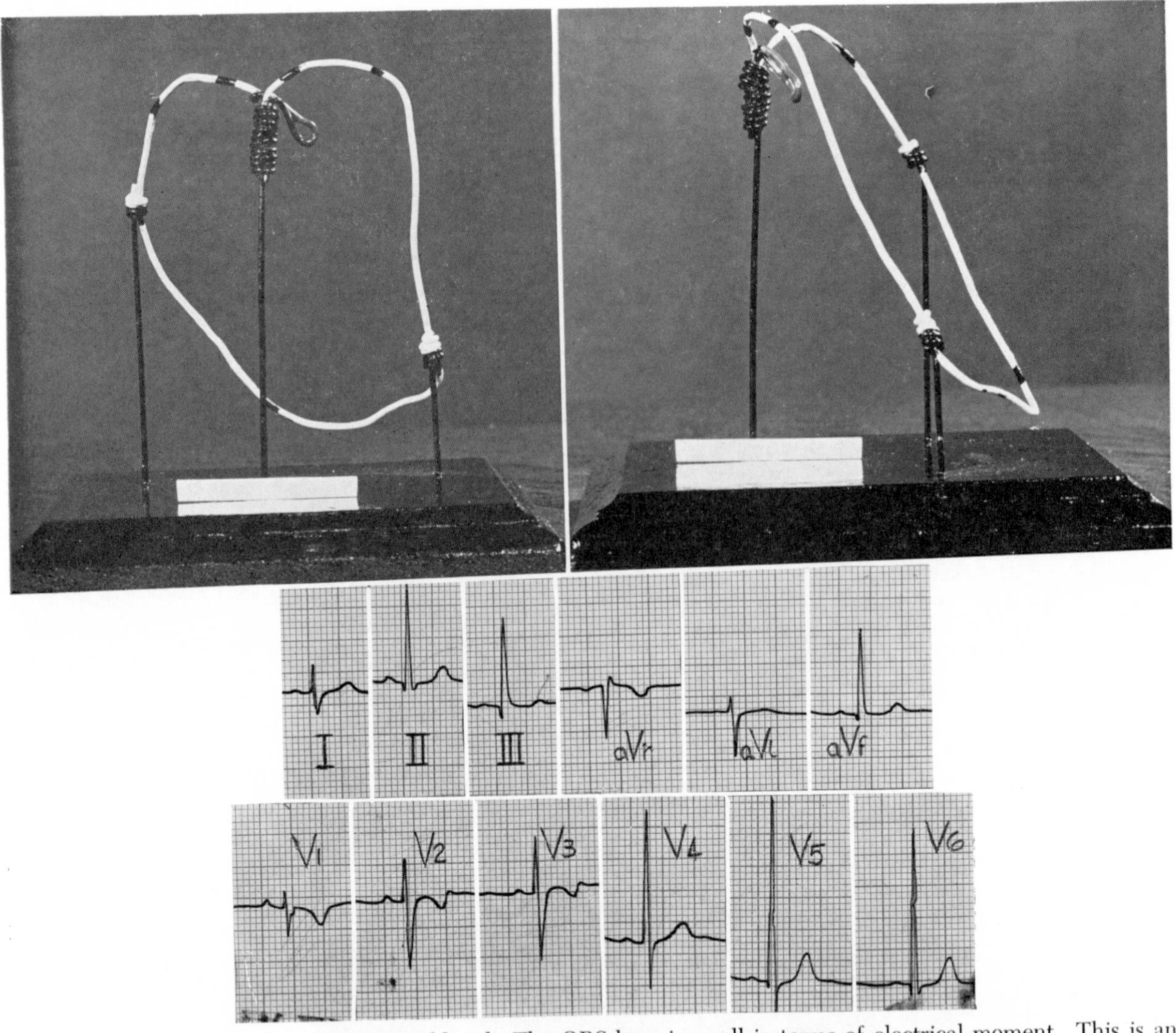

Figure 91. The VCG of an eight year old girl. The QRS loop is small in terms of electrical moment. This is an excellent example of small QRS amplitude when expressed in terms of electrode placement. The QRS amplitude on the routing ECG is not expressed in terms of electrode placement and the QRS amplitude therefore bears no relation to the true size of the small heart of this 56 pound child. The small P loop is directed posteriorly and obscured by the larger T loop. The T loop is directed posteriorly on the VCG and is manifested by an inverted T wave in V1, V2, and V3. This is the juvenile pattern. The spatial VCG suggests that the apex of the heart may be pointed backward in such examples.

The vectorcardiogram provides a clear demonstration of the influence of respiration. The expiratory VCG consistently is the largest. At the onset of inspiration there is marked decrease in size of the last half of the QRS loop representing the left ventricle and slight increase in the anterior segment. When the breath is held in deep inspiration the left ventricular component momentarily increases with the surge of blood from the lungs into the left ventricle but there is an over-all decrease in the loop consistent with decreased stroke volume (this is most marked in complete valsalva). On expiration the VCG is momentarily larger than during quiet breathing. The temporal changes in the QRS cycle do not permit the simple explanation of change in cardiac position due to excursion of the diaphragm (Fig. 98).

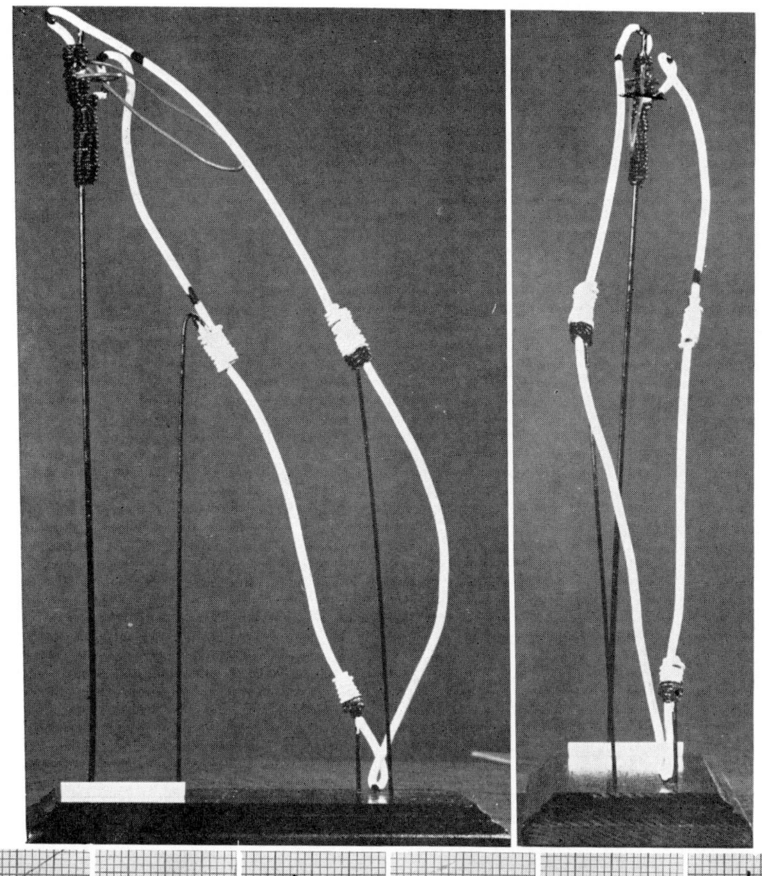

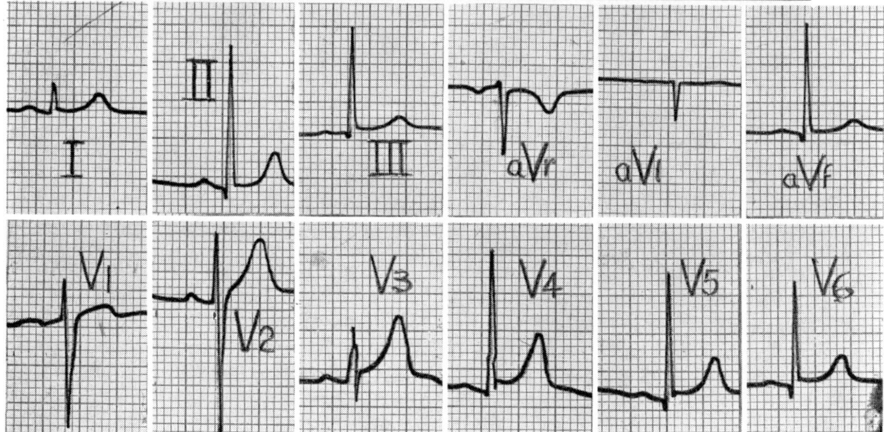

Figure 92. The VCG of an eighteen year old healthy male. The initial upward course of the QRS loop creates an initial R wave in aVr. The QRS loop remains open indicating a force is still active at the completion of excitation. This is the same as the elevation of the ST segment seen in Leads I, II, III, aVf, and V2 through V6. The QRS loop continues directly into the T loop. The P loop is very small and directed nearly straight to the left.

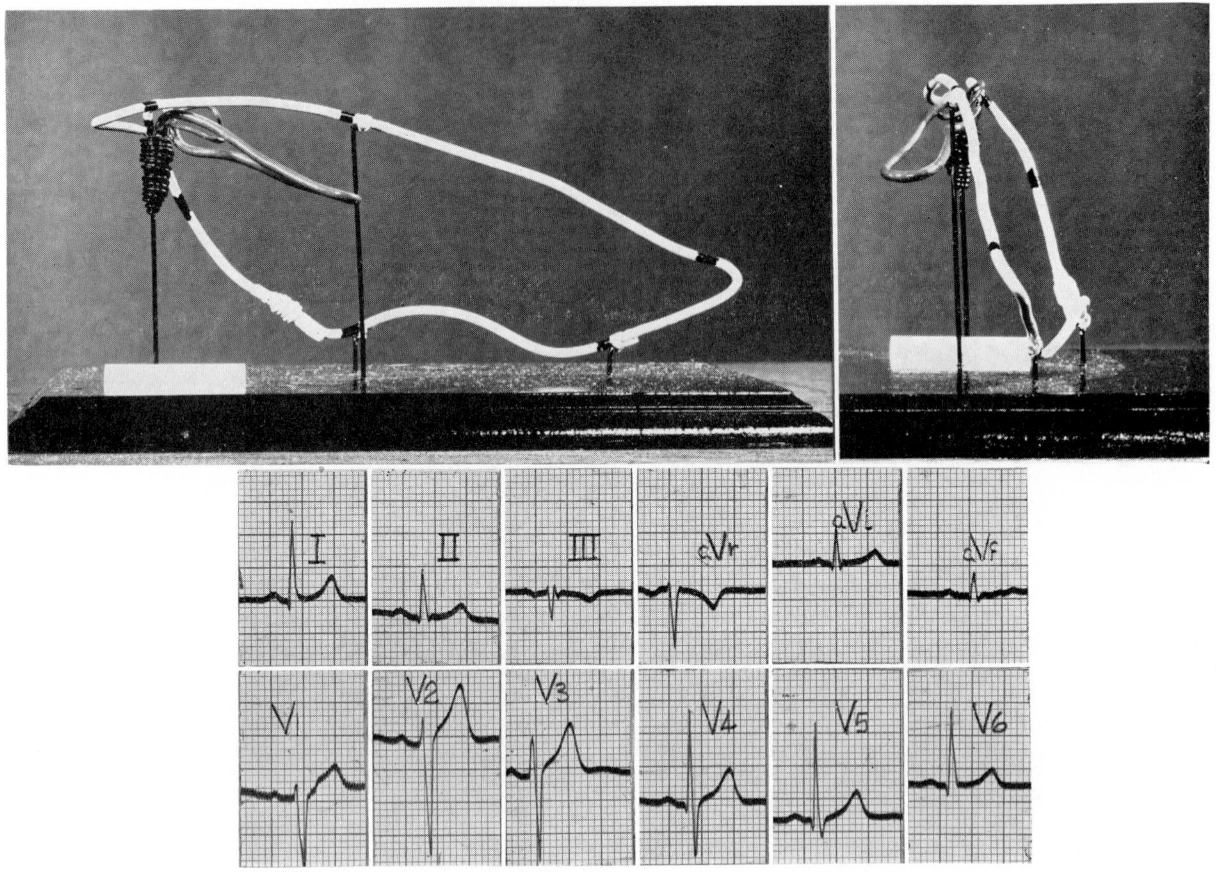

Figure 93. The VCG of a forty-three year old man. The QRS loop is intermediate in location. The initial rightward course of the QRS loop corresponds to the initial Q wave in Lead I and the initial R wave in Lead III. The subsequent leftward QRS pathway writes an R wave in Lead I and an S wave in Lead III. When the QRS pathway descends it enters the positive zone of Lead III creating an R′ wave. The terminal QRS pathway is directed upward to such a degree that a terminal S′ wave is inscribed in Lead III.

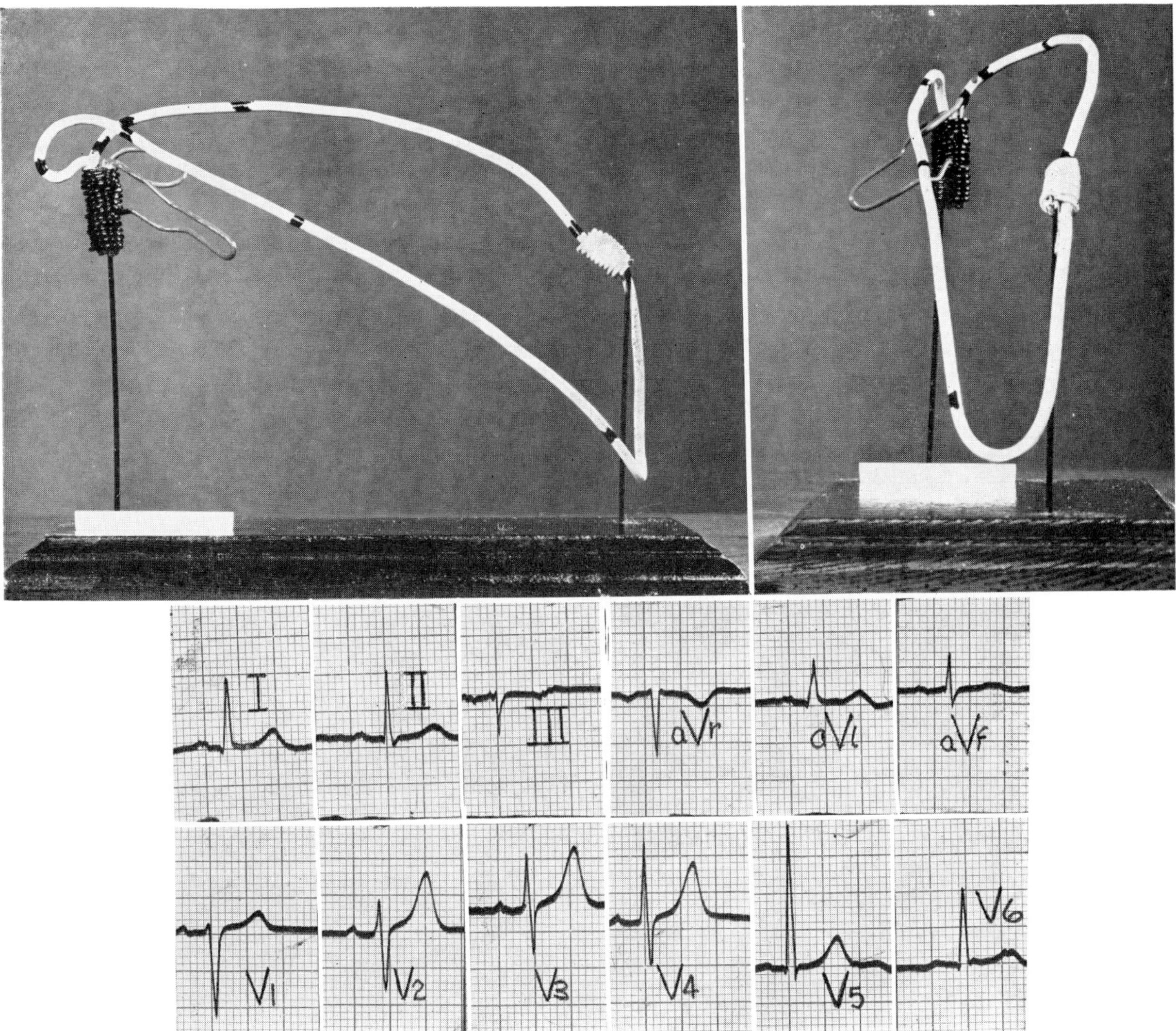

Figure 94. An intermediate VCG in a normal forty year old man. The QRS pathway is first directed to the right and downward (Q wave in Lead I and embryonic R wave in Lead III). As the pathway is directed upward a tiny S wave is inscribed in Lead III. The QRS pathway continues to the left and is the inferior limb of the main QRS loop. It invades only a little way into the positive zone of Lead III creating an R′ wave of very low amplitude. The terminal QRS pathway is well within the negative zone of Lead III creating a more prominent S′ wave. The chief difference in this VCG from Fig. 93 is that the main terminal QRS pathway is above the main initial large QRS pathway, thus there is no R′ wave following the main S wave in Lead III. The initial R wave in the V leads becomes progressively larger as the V lead axis becomes more leftward. Compare the configuration of Lead I and V6.

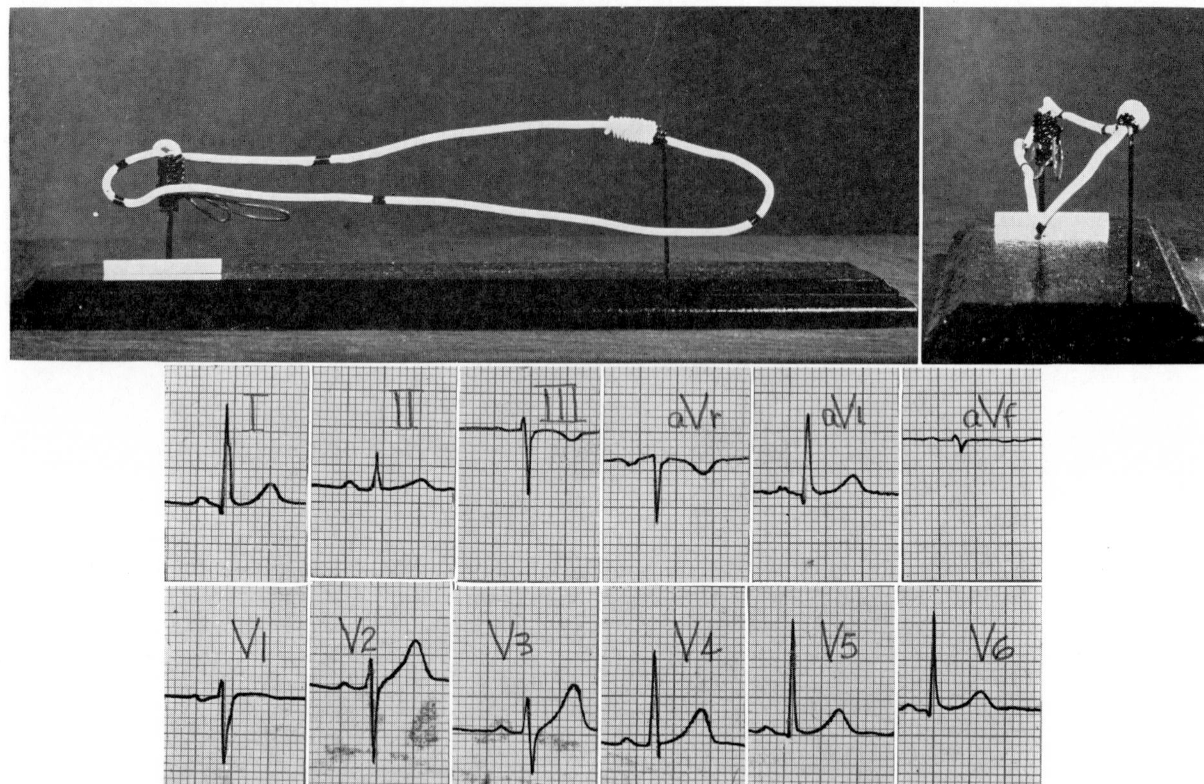

Figure 95. A VCG with horizontal orientation. The QRS loop is narrow and nearly perpendicular to aVf. This accounts for the low amplitude and diphasic character of the QRS loop in that lead. The loop is also narrow in the sagittal view corresponding to the low QRS amplitude in V2. The area of such long narrow loops is quite small. Calculations based on the enclosed area are meaningless. In such examples only the correct principles of the polygon sides (length of QRS pathway) can be expected to reflect the magnitude of electrical activity. The P loop as usual is smaller than the T loop.

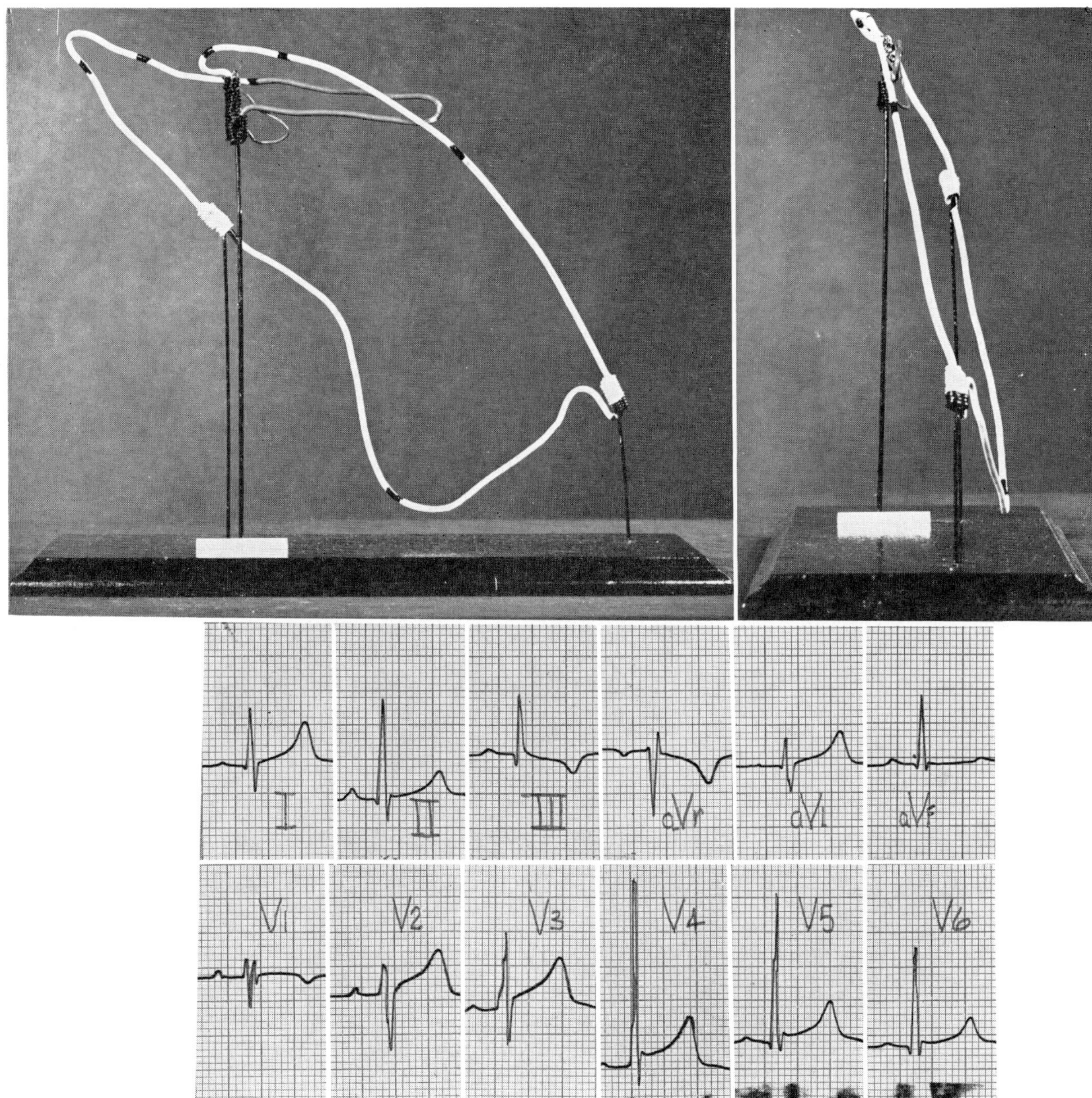

Figure 96. The VCG of a twenty-seven year old Olympic athlete. The qRS configuration of Lead I can readily be extracted from the frontal plane. Regard the 5 cm. standardization to appreciate the tremendous size of the VCG. The marked increase in QRS amplitude is lost in the routine ECG. The subject has a resting pulse rate of 44 per min. with necessarily increased stroke volume. The ST interval creates an open QRS loop. The T loop is large and normally directed. The smaller P loop is clearly evident.

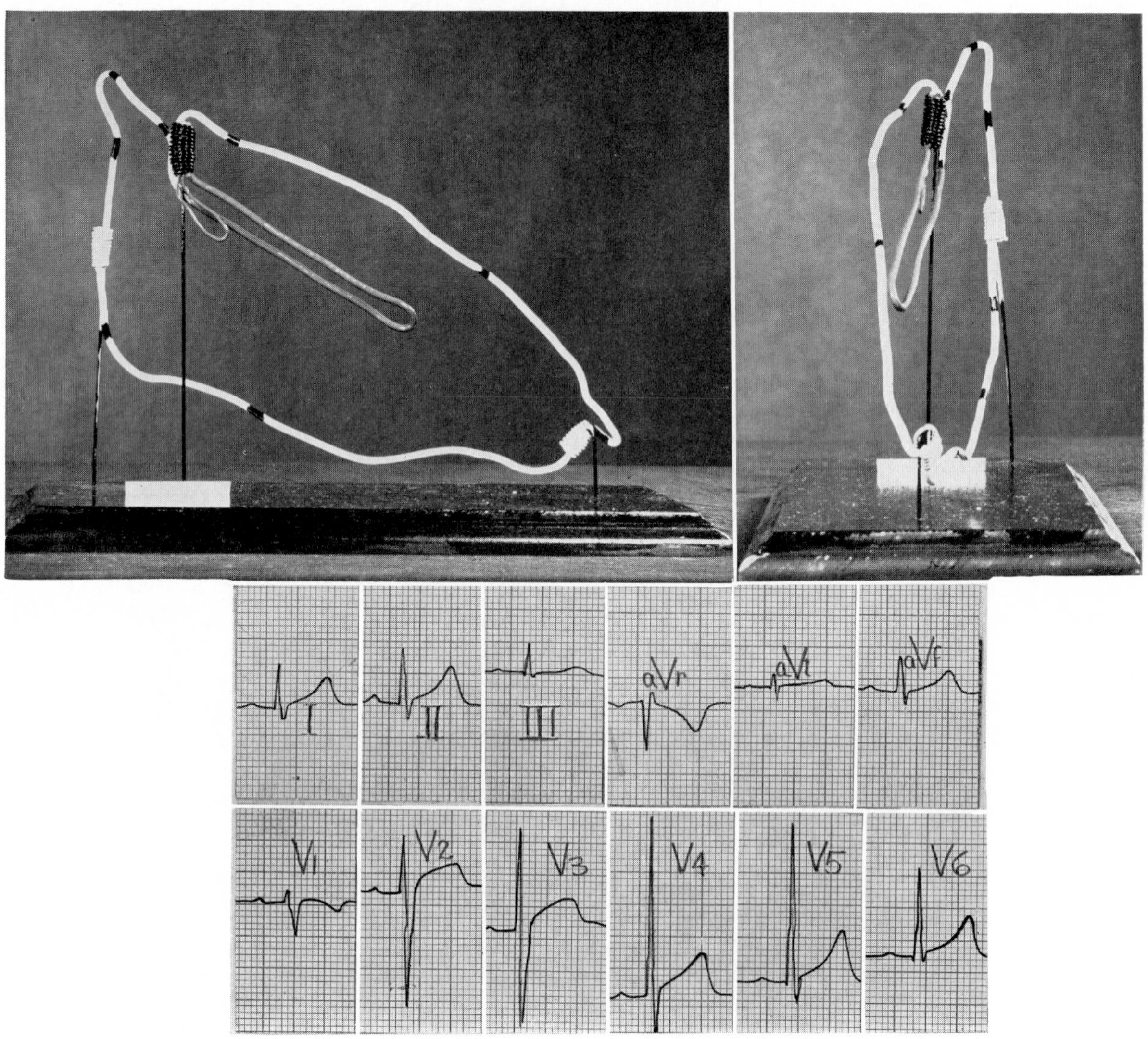

Figure 97. The VCG of a thirty-seven year old Olympic athlete, pulse 46, B.P. 92/52. The large QRS loop is clearly evident associated with a large T loop and smaller P loop. The QRS loop is open.

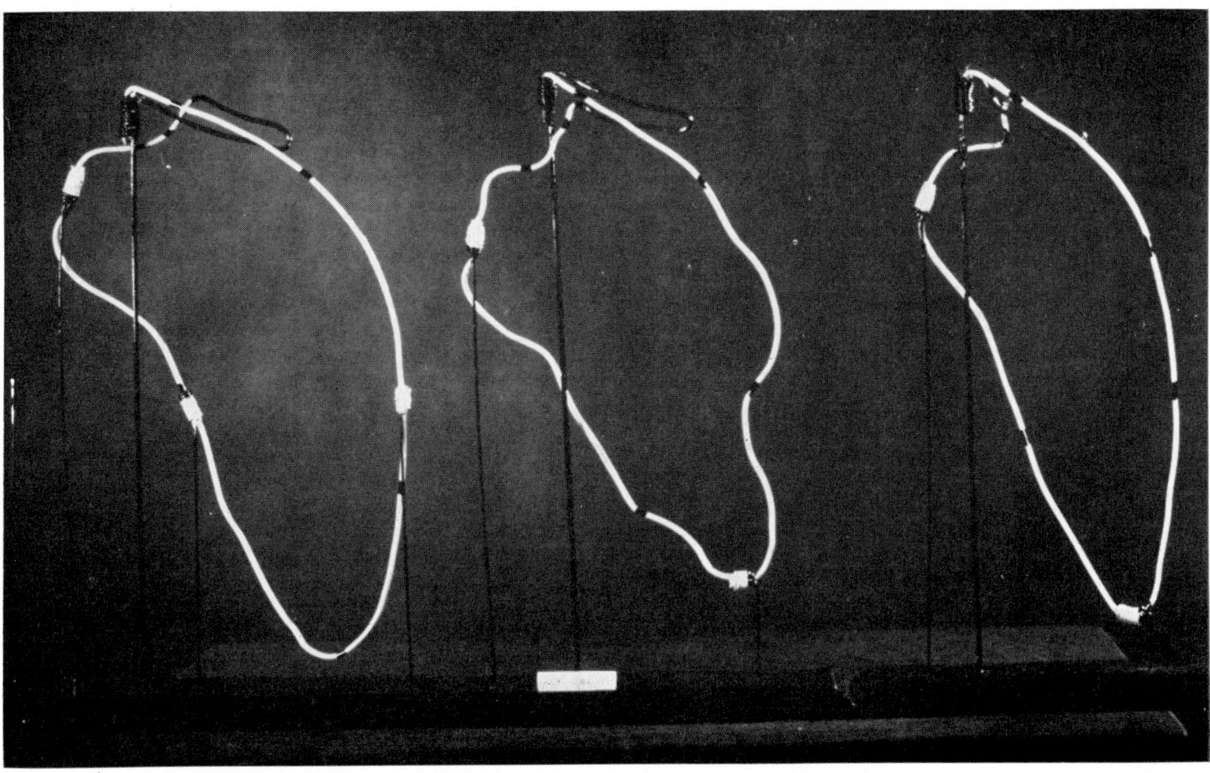

Figure 98. The VCG shows marked changes during the respiratory cycle. The above models are all of the same individual. On the left the subject is in expiration. The center model represents the early phase of inspiration. The model on the right shows the increase in size of the VCG that occurs while holding the breath in full inspiration, despite the fact the lungs are at maximum inflation. Note the absence of rightward shift of the VCG and the selective changes in the last half of QRS pathway on early inspiration.

IX

Cardiac Enlargement

ATRIAL ENLARGEMENT

ATRIAL ENLARGEMENT is manifested by an increase in duration or amplitude of the P wave. It is not possible to detect which atrial chamber is enlarged from the routine electrocardiogram. However, there is a tendency for a more leftward P loop or P axis with left atrial enlargement and a more vertical loop with right atrial enlargement (Figs. 99 and 100).

LEFT VENTRICULAR ENLARGEMENT

As the left ventricle enlarges, the length of time required for completion of a confluent wave front of excitation is increased. This is caused by the increase in endocardial area to be excited, or directly related to ventricular dilatation. This factor can increase the time required for excitation (increased QRS duration) without significant increase in wall thickness.

Dilatation of the left ventricle increases its surface area and consequently increases the size of the excitation wave front. This is manifested by increased QRS amplitude, increased index of maximum potential and increased potential seconds. The septum remains as a 60° arc of the ventricular cone. Elongation of the ventricle increases the septal area (in relation to the base). The increased septal component opens the spatial QRS loop creating a prominent posterior component during the last half of the QRS cycle. The open loop is characteristic of ventricular dilatation and elongation. Opening of the loop cannot be determined on the routine ECG. It is related to the amplitude and difference in time between the S wave in V2 and the R wave in V6.

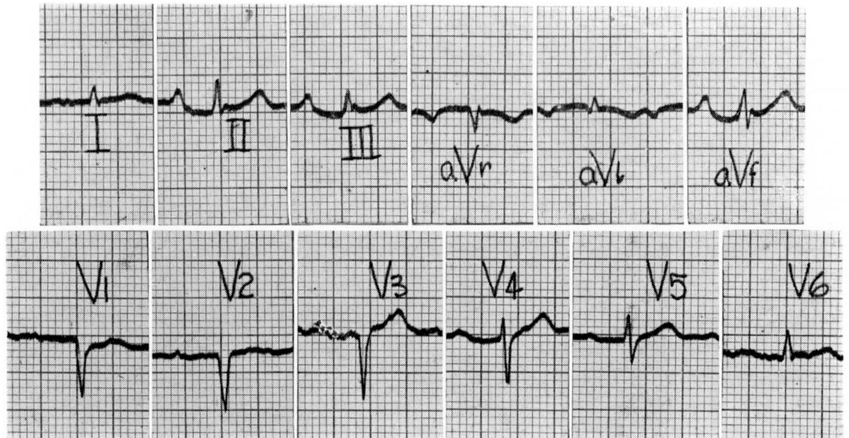

Figure 99. The ECG of advanced pulmonary emphysema. The PR interval is prolonged to .24 sec. The mean P vector is +90° with an isoelectric P interval in Lead I. The mean QRS axis is +60°. Note the low amplitude of the QRS complexes throughout the record. The distinctive features are the comparatively large P waves with vertical P axis and the very small QRS amplitude.

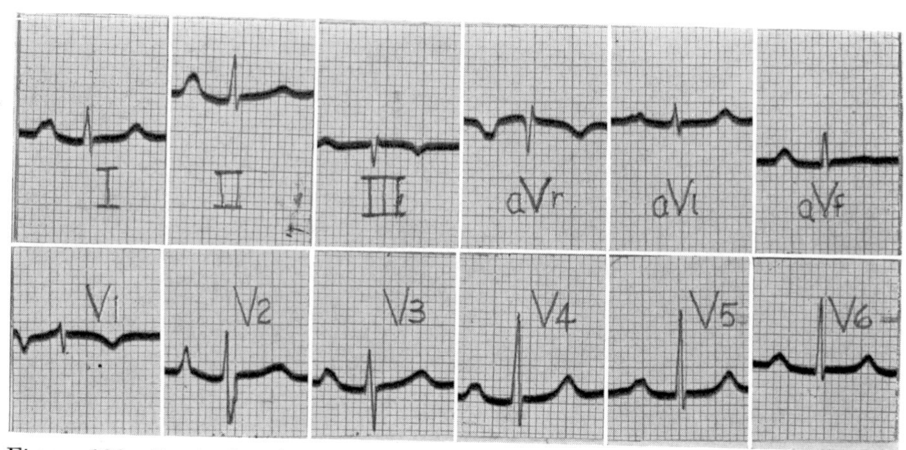

Figure 100. P mitral. This is an example of mitral stenosis and insufficiency. PR interval .26 sec.; increased P amplitude; P axis +45°; comparatively small QRS amplitude; mean QRS axis +15°. The distinctive feature is the large P waves in Lead I and II.

Amplitude is often misleading when measured by the routine ECG due to electrode distance and lead length. Whenever the sum of the amplitude of the QRS complexes in Leads V6, V2 and aVf exceeds 5 millivolts, the question of dilatation should be considered. A prominent S wave in V2 is a frequent finding in left ventricular hypertrophy.

Generalized dilatation may be manifested by increased voltage. The increased magnitude seen in the presence of a normally slow heart is such an example. There is an increase in amplitude in both the R wave and S wave in V2. In isolated left ventricular hypertrophy the R wave is normal or diminished in amplitude whereas the S wave is increased in size. The increase in voltage caused by uncomplicated left ventricular hypertrophy affects chiefly the last half of the excitation cycle or that portion dominated by the left ventricle.

The value of converting measurements to terms of electrical moment is evident in comparing such a vectorcardiogram in a child, a normal adult, and in the presence of hypertrophy (Fig. 101). It is known that the child's heart is small and the relative size difference can be appreciated in this manner.

Increase in wall thickness increases the QRS duration and the potential seconds. The QRS duration becomes more significant as an index of wall thickness in the absence of dilatation (normal QRS amplitude).

Ventricular recovery is altered in the presence of left ventricular hypertrophy. With increased wall thickness the time required for transmission of the wave front of recovery to the surface is increased. The early endocardial recovery at the apex creates a wave front before arrival at the epicardial surface. This wave front directs forces towards the recovered endocardial tissues or towards the base. The apical endocardial recovery creates an ST segment depression in those leads with an upright QRS complex. The degree of depression depends upon the degree of wall thickness.

It is interesting to note that physiological enlargement as seen in the athlete is often accompanied by ST segment changes. These, however, are due to a vector directed parallel to the QRS vector and are associated with early recovery of the right ventricle and apical regions throughout the thin wall.

With increased wall thickness the conical wave front of recovery develops steeper walls or a cylindrical shape. This diminishes the magnitude of the T loop and T waves. Progressive wall thickening results in an everted conical wave front throughout the endocardial shell. At this point the T vector is directed opposite the QRS vector or creates a wide spatial QRS-T

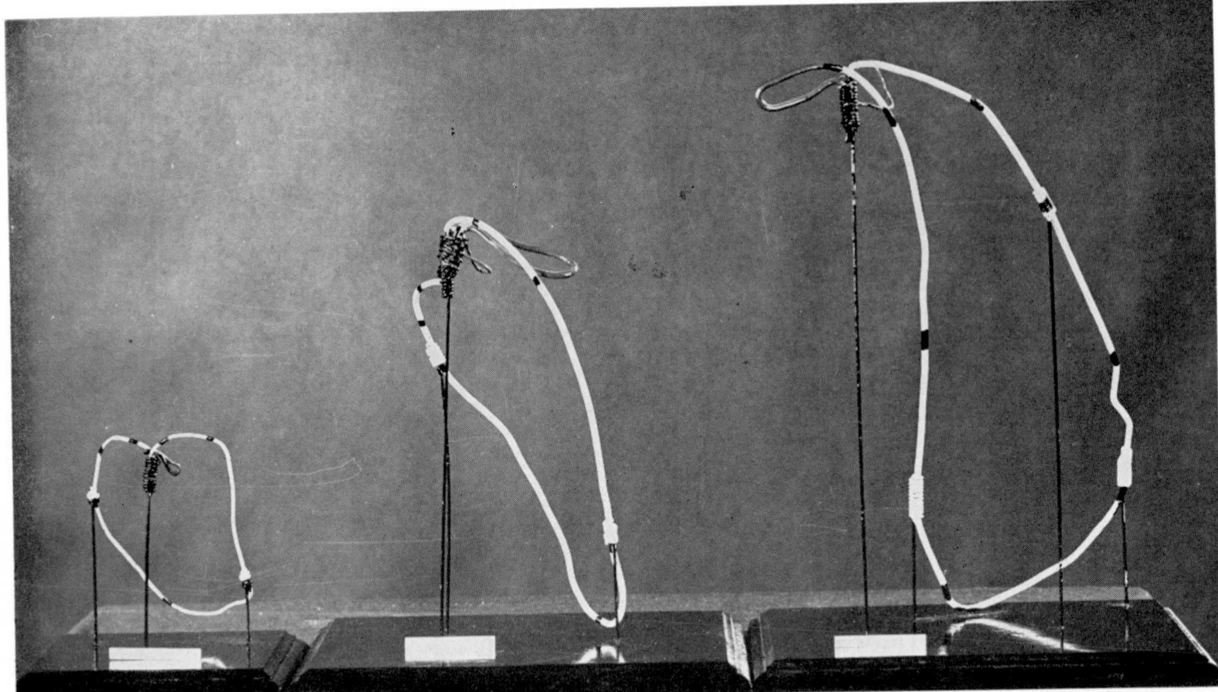

Figure 101. Three VCG models constructed to the same scale (see standardization bar). The left model is a fifty-six pound child. The center model is a normal twenty-two year old 155 pound male. The model on the right is that of a twenty-one year old female, at 120 pounds with congenital aortic stenosis and marked left ventricular enlargement. The difference in cardiac size is unquestioned clinically and the difference in the VCG model size is obvious.

angle, the T loop is opposite the QRS loop, the QRS complexes are upright with inverted T waves. The inverted T wave becomes progressively larger after this stage.

The increased time required for excitation and recovery causes an increase in the QT interval. Physiological enlargement, which is chiefly dilatation, is associated with a large, normally directed T loop (Fig. 102).

Left ventricular hypertrophy may be present with vertical intermediate or left electrical axis (Figs. 103 and 104). Marked left axis is more apt to occur with elongation of the ventricle in association with other physical factors. A high incidence of angina, previous infarction and conduction defects occurs in subjects with an electrical axis farther left than –30°.

Left ventricular hypertrophy causes:*

1) Increased QRS duration (increased potential seconds).

2) Increased QRS amplitude (increased index of maximum potential).

3) An ST vector directed away from the QRS vector. Physiological dilatation creates an ST vector parallel to the QRS and T vectors.

4) Decreased T vector magnitude. Physiological dilatation increases T vector magnitude.

5) Isoelectric T waves.

6) Inverted T waves with a wide QRS-T angle. Physiological dilatation is associated with a normal directed T wave.

7) Increased QT interval.

RIGHT VENTRICULAR ENLARGEMENT

Enlargement of the right ventricle creates particularly complicated electrocardiographic

*There is a wide difference of opinion amongst authorities regarding what is left ventricular hypertrophy by the ECG. This is hardly surprising since the important factors of magnitude are not considered (electrode distance and lead length), the difference in opinion in determination and use of the so called intrinsicoid deflection, the failure to use the sides of the polygon principle to evaluate magnitude and the absence of any correlation of QRS magnitude to cardiac rate.

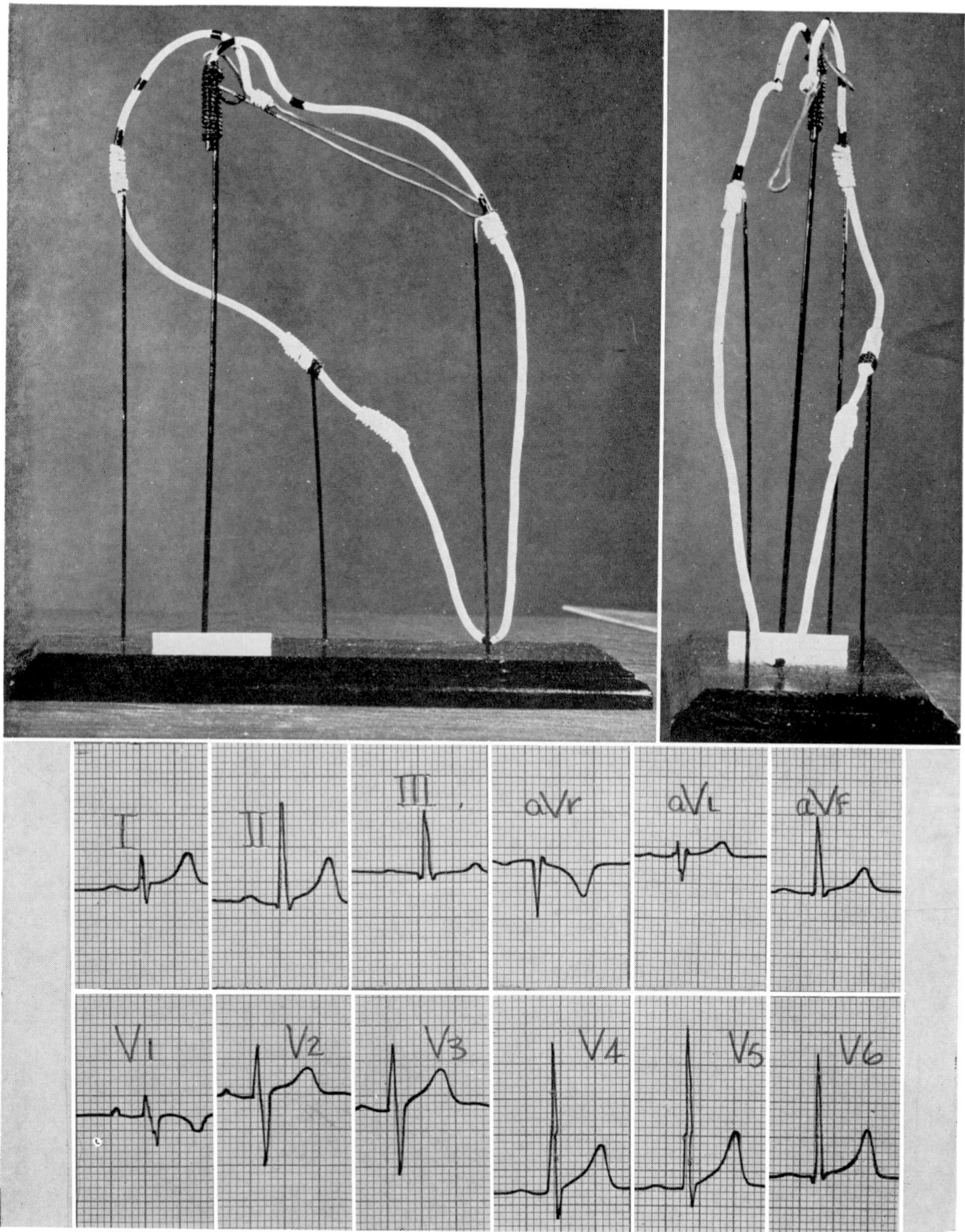

Figure 102. The VCG of an Olympic athlete. The large normally directed T loop is characteristic of physiological dilatation. The ST interval is manifested by a normally directed ST force. There is an overall enlargement of the entire QRS loop as one would expect from generalized dilatation. Thus the R wave in V2 is large compared to the S wave. Contrast this to the R/S ratio in hypertrophy due to selective increased work of the left ventricle in the subsequent figures.

manifestations. In addition to a simple consideration of chamber size and wall thickness, there is the problem of change in position of the left ventricle secondary to right ventricular dilatation.

Simple uncomplicated right ventricular dilatation pushes the left ventricle posteriorly (Fig. 105). This simple maneuver causes the terminal events of left ventricular excitation to describe a spatial pathway to the right and posterior. It requires only a small backward shift of the apex to accomplish this effect. The left ventricle then creates a larger S wave in Lead I with a vertical or rightward mean QRS axis. There is an S wave in Lead V2. The terminal rightward pathway may describe an R′ wave at V1.

As long as the left ventricle is the last to complete excitation, the S wave in Lead I cannot be ascribed to the right ventricle. When the right ventricle dominates the terminal excitation, there will be little, if any, S wave in Lead V2.

Dilatation of the right ventricle causes prolongation of the time required to form a confluent wave front of excitation. This prolongation in

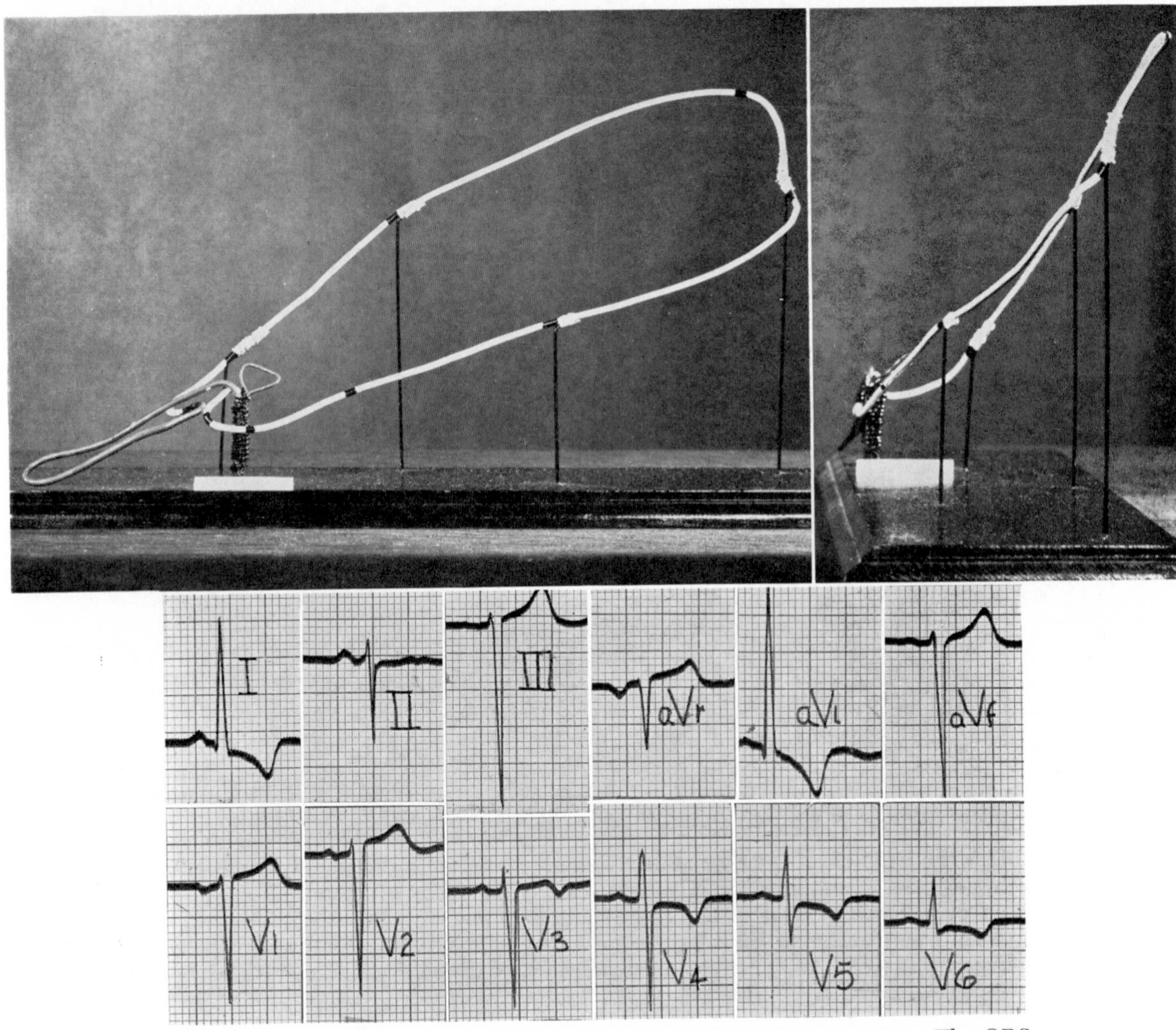

Figure 103. The VCG of left ventricular hypertrophy in hypertension. The QRS amplitude is markedly increased. The QRS loop is directed backward. The large T loop is directed opposite the QRS loop. Note the ST interval is directed parallel to the T loop. The V leads are recorded at half standard.

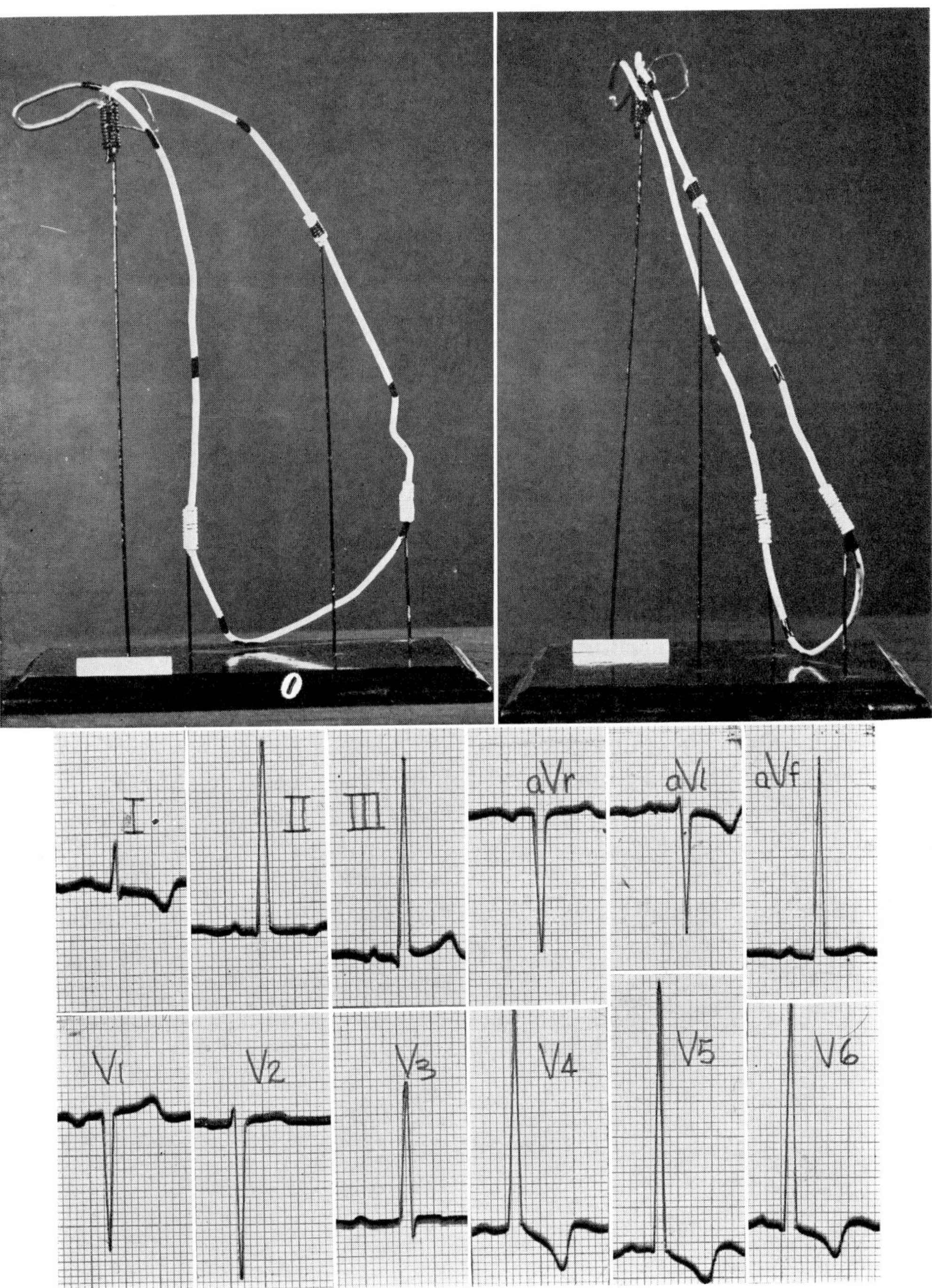

Figure 104. The VCG of twenty-one year old case of aortic stenosis. The QRS loop is vertical but again chiefly posterior in its orientation. The T loop is comparatively smaller than the previous example and is directed opposite the QRS loop. The P loop is directed backward. Leads V2 and V3 are recorded at half standard.

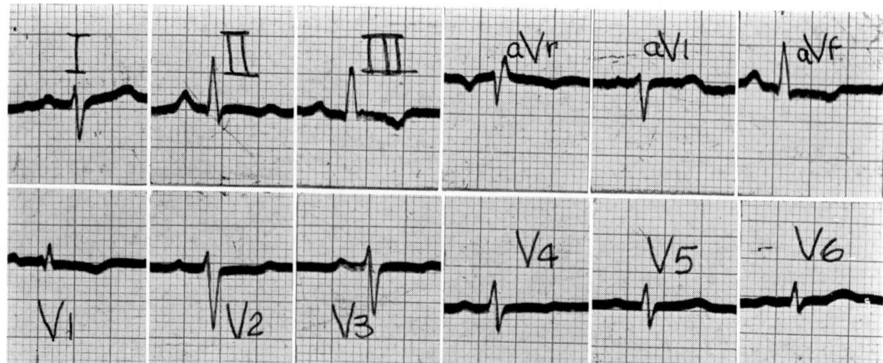

Figure 105. Right ventricular dilatation with a mean QRS axis of +105°. The terminal S wave in V2 and Lead I represent the terminal forces of left ventricle. An S wave in Lead I due to the right ventricle would not have an S wave in V2.

time of excitation may allow the right ventricle to create a large force during the period normally occupied by left ventricular excitation alone. This opposite force diminishes the QRS amplitude and the index of maximum potential.

The thicker base may be sufficiently delayed in activation to create a late R wave from the right ventricle alone. In this case, right ventricular hypertrophy resembles the electrocardiographic pattern of right bundle branch block (Fig. 106). It differs from bundle branch block in that its index of maximum potential is usually less.

Right ventricular dilatation may cause:

1) Increased QRS duration.

2) Decreased index of maximum potential.

3) Right axis shift of mean QRS axis manifested by a prominent S wave in Leads I and V6, terminal R′ wave in V1 and terminal R in Lead III.

4) Delay in activation of the base with complicated conduction resembling bundle branch block.

When right ventricular dilatation is associated with increased wall thickness there is further prolongation in its activation. The prolonged period of activation may maintain a larger wave front in the right ventricle than in the left. This creates right ventricular dominance of excitation. As left ventricular activation is completed the right ventricular force directs the spatial pathway anterior. If right ventricular dominance is maintained, the entire pathway is displaced anterior to the point of origin.

In this instance the rightward axis with terminal S wave in Leads I and V6 is due to the

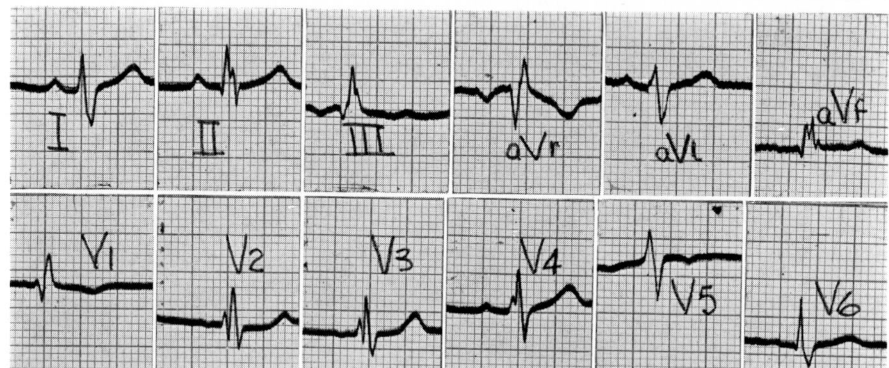

Figure 106. An ECG of an adult with anomalous pulmonary venous drainage into the right atrium. The apparent right bundle branch block may disappear following surgical correction of the cause for right ventricular hypertrophy in such cases.

right ventricle. The QRS complex in V2 is chiefly positive with little or no S wave. These findings are most often seen in congenital lesions placing the increased work chiefly on the right ventricle, e.g., atrial septal defect and pulmonary stenosis. Since the right heart is larger at birth, the disproportion persists and the left ventricle never has an opportunity to exceed the size of the right ventricle.

Mitral stenosis with advanced right ventricular hypertrophy can develop an anterior loop with a completely positive QRS at V2. Left ventricular atrophy may contribute to the imbalance. When the left ventricle remains of normal thickness or if other complications are present, the S wave in V2 will be more prominent. Decrease in the index of maximum potential is almost constant in the presence of

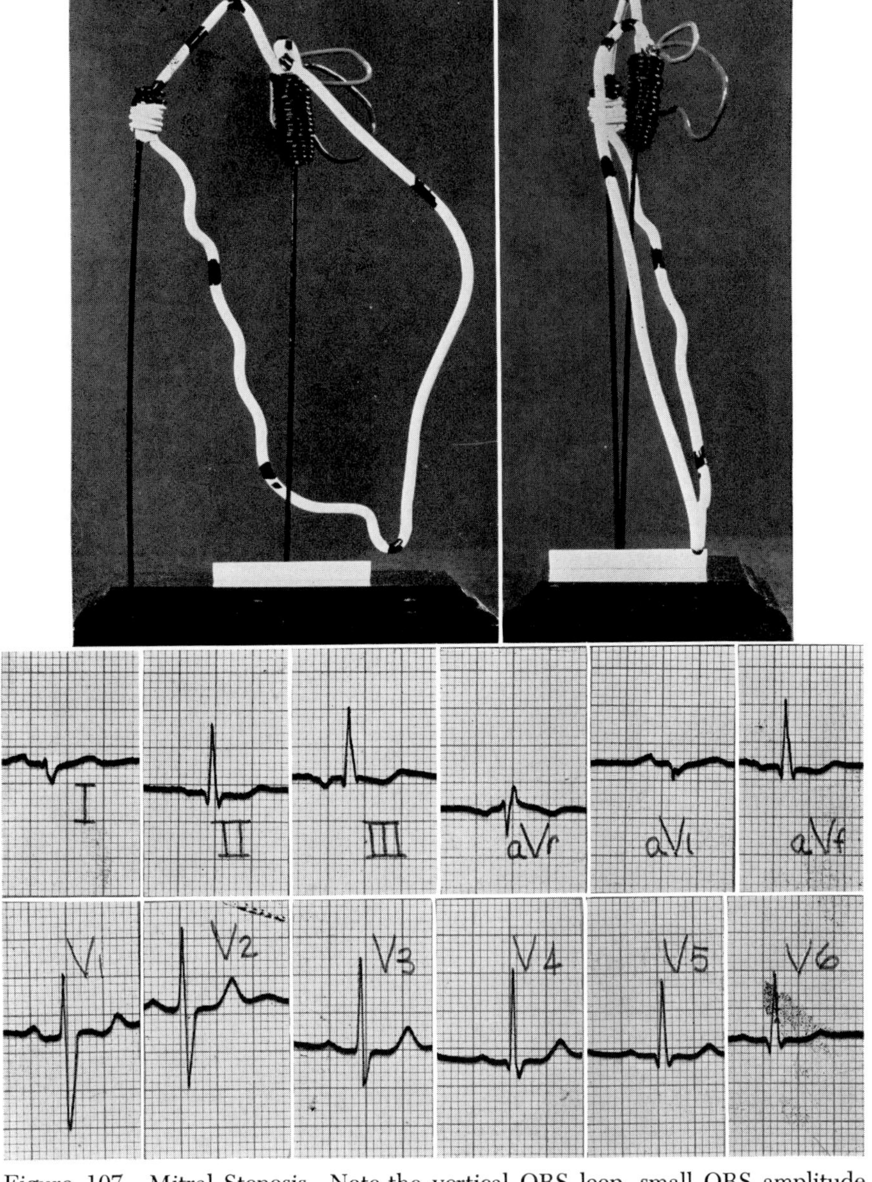

Figure 107. Mitral Stenosis. Note the vertical QRS loop, small QRS amplitude and prominent early anterior pathway of the QRS loop (prominent R wave in V2). The P loop is the most leftward loop (mean P axis —15°). The leftward P loop (left atrium) and vertical QRS axis suggests mitral stenosis.

significant mitral stenosis. The possibility of muscular damage due to rheumatic activity could be an associated factor (Figs. 107 and 108).

As right ventricular hypertrophy ensues, becoming the dominant ventricle with a thick wall, it effects ventricular recovery much as does left ventricular hypertrophy. The T vector rotates away from the QRS forces widening the mean spatial QRS-T angle.

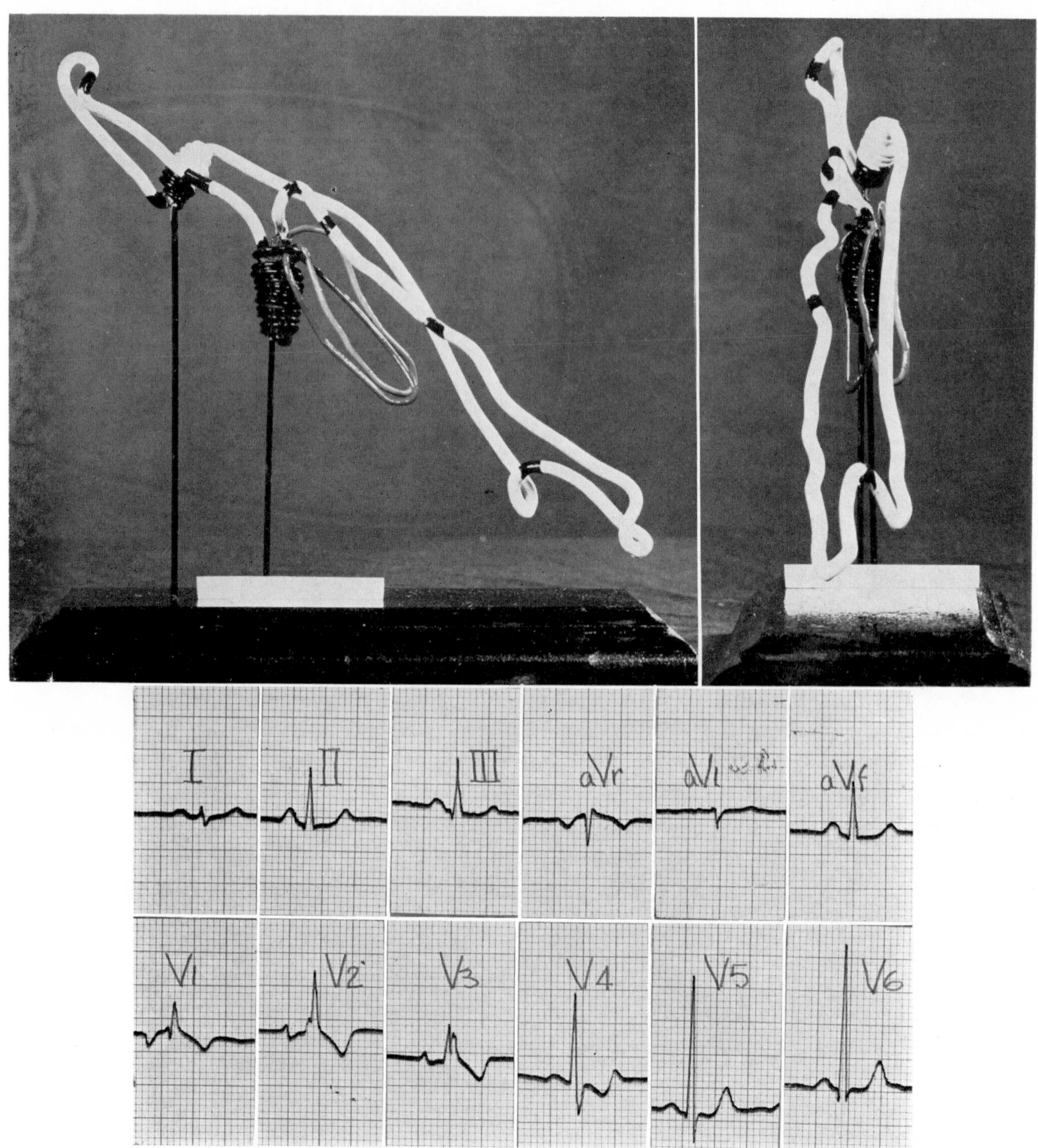

Figure 108. Advanced Mitral Stenosis: The small QRS loop is directed anteriorly (R wave in V2). The P loop is approximately as large as the T loop.

X

Conduction Defects

LEFT BUNDLE BRANCH BLOCK

The simplest form of left bundle branch block is a single localized interruption of the left bundle, with the rest of the endocardial conduction system intact. Due to the block in the left bundle the excitation impulse passes through the right bundle from the AV node. This causes excitation to begin at the right endocardial region at the septal area (Fig. 109).

Activation of the right septal surface creates a force directed posterior and slightly to the left, (.005 sec.). When the right ventricular cone of activation is complete (.02 sec.) the resultant force is more leftward and commonly posterior. Excitation spreads outward from all regions. The free wall of the right ventricle gradually completes activation causing the instantaneous vector to be directed even more posteriorly. The excitation wave reaches the endocardial surface of the left ventricle at its thinnest region at .04 sec. As soon as the impulse reaches the left ventricle, rapid endocardial excitation occurs. As the left ventricular cone becomes confluent the instantaneous vector moves leftward, retaining its posterior direction. By .06 sec., the wave front is the 300° arc, left ventricular cone. The magnitude of the vector gradually diminishes to zero as excitation proceeds to completion.

The order of excitation in left bundle branch block commonly creates an early posterior pathway. The normal loop creates an early anterior pathway. Thus the loops of left bundle branch block are usually just opposite in direction to the normal loop.

The duration of excitation is prolonged to 0.12 sec. The free wall of the left ventricle normally requires 0.08 sec. for excitation. The free wall does not receive activation until the impulse crosses the septum which requires 0.04 sec. in the presence of complete block. Thus the delay in septal activation is responsible for the prolonged excitation.

Recovery begins at the right ventricular region. The formation of an endocardial wave front near the apex creates a force directed toward the base of the right ventricle. As recovery ensues, the free wall of the right ventricle completes activation. The septum undergoes recovery from both sides, thus its force is small or non existent. The left ventricular free wall recovers from the endocardial region. The resultant vector of the wave front is directed toward the septum and left ventricular base (Fig. 110). Recovery of the right ventricle prevents the QRS loop from closing and subsequent recovery creates a spatial pathway opposite the pathway of excitation.

If one projects the instantaneous vectors of the spatial pathway created by left bundle branch block on the lead coordinates, the pattern of left bundle branch block is created. Since the QRS loop is directed posterior, the QRS complexes in V1 and V2 are commonly negative deflections and the leftward course creates a positive QRS complex in Leads I and V6. The onset of right ventricular recovery creates a force opposite the QRS loop or an ST segment depression in those leads with an upright QRS complex. The T loop is opposite the QRS loop and creates a negative T wave in leads with an upright QRS complex (Fig. 111).

The characteristics of left bundle branch

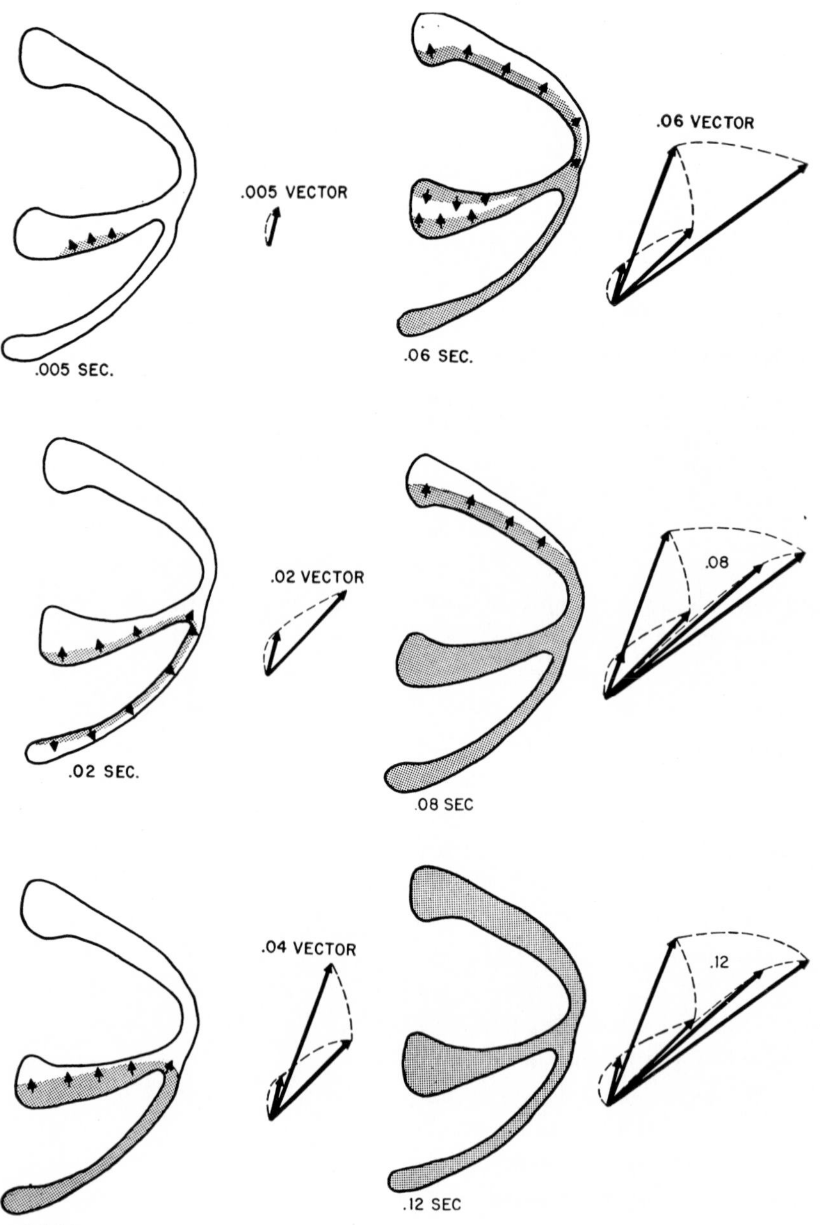

Figure 109. Order of excitation in left bundle branch block.

block noted on the routine ECG are:

1) QRS duration of 0.12 sec. or more.

2) Upright QRS complexes in Lead I and V6.

3) ST segment depression in Lead I and V6 or an ST vector opposite the mean QRS vector.

4) Inverted T waves in leads with upright QRS complexes, i.e., a mean T vector directed opposite the mean QRS vector.

In the event there is loss or absence of additional specialized conduction tissue in the left ventricle, activation through the left ventricle will be slowed. In its greatest extreme the entire left ventricle could require activation by slow muscle spread. This would greatly prolong the QRS duration beyond 0.12 sec.

The clinical significance of left bundle branch block depends upon its cause. It may be caused by arteriosclerotic heart disease, or myocarditis. In very rare instances it is thought to be congenital in origin. Left bundle branch block

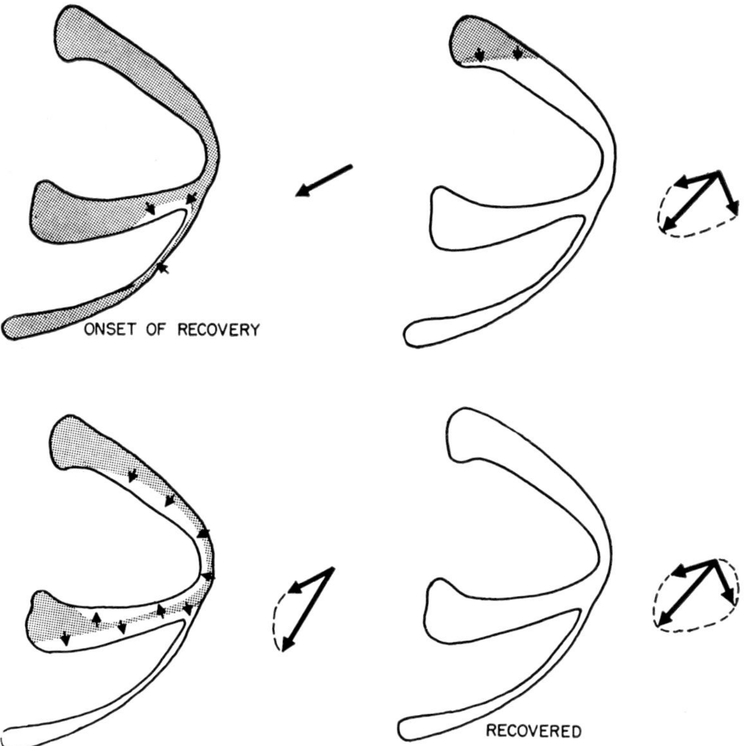

Figure 110. Order of recovery in left bundle branch block.

without cardiac disease is almost nonexistent in children.

RIGHT BUNDLE BRANCH BLOCK

Whenever septal activation is accomplished from only one side, it will require twice the usual length of time. When the right bundle is blocked, activation begins normally at the left endocardial surface and forms a normal left ventricular conical wave front. Right ventricular activation begins when this wave front crosses the septum. The thick base of the right ventricle is the last to be activated. The terminal force is to the right and anterior (Fig. 112).

The initial forces of excitation are created by normal left ventricular activation and are manifested by an anterior pathway. There may be a very small, short duration, force directed to the right, with the onset of septal activation. The remainder of the early pathway is leftward. The terminal pathway is rightward and anterior. The initial and terminal anterior direction of the forces creates an R R′ wave over the anterior precordium at V1 and V2. The QRS complex at V1 and V2 may be entirely positive. The terminal rightward forces creates a terminal S wave in Lead I and usually a terminal R wave in Lead III (Figs. 113, 114 and 115).

Recovery proceeds normally from apex to base creating a force directed toward the apex. Thus there is a normal upright T wave in Lead I. This has lead to the observation that the T was upright in the lead with the terminal S wave (Lead I).

The characteristics of right bundle branch block are:

1) QRS duration of 0.11 sec. or more.

2) Terminal S wave in Lead I and terminal R wave in V1, (a terminal right anterior vector).

3) There may be T wave changes secondary to the change in order of activation.

Right bundle branch block seems to be more common than left bundle branch block in otherwise normal children. Its presence does not demand a bad prognosis. The problem is to detect underlying heart disease if any. Right ven-

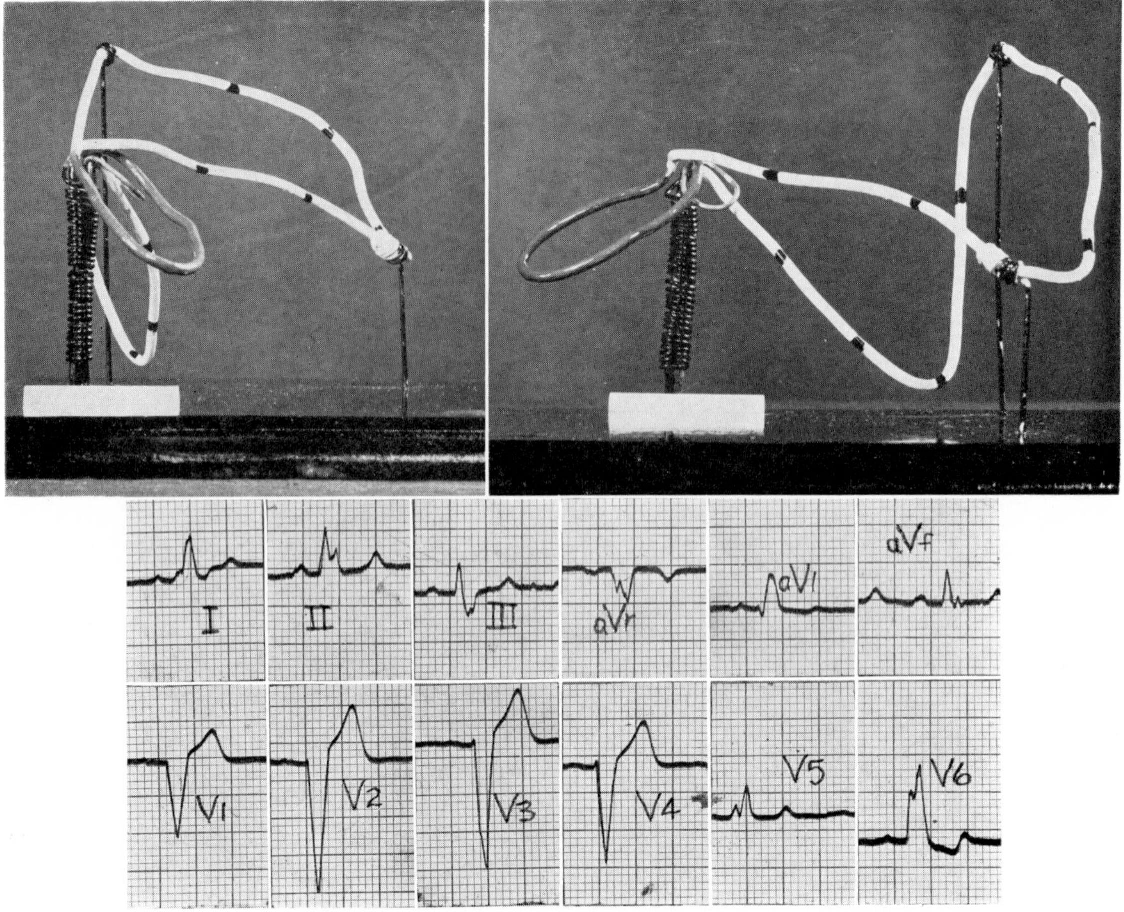

Figure 111. A thirty year old pilot with complete left bundle branch block of undetermined origin. Correlate the model with the earlier example of the order of excitation and recovery, then project model on lead coordinates to construct 12 lead electrocardiograms.

tricular dilatation and hypertrophy often creates similar or indistinguishable findings. The differentiation of right bundle branch block from right ventricular hypertrophy is not entirely satisfactory by current methods.

THE S_1 S_2 S_3 PATTERN

A frequent finding in young people is the presence of a terminal S wave in Leads I, II, and III (Fig. 116). This means the terminal force of excitation must be directed toward the right shoulder. In some instances this is associated with an rSr′ at V1 and in other instances with a terminal broad S wave at V1. This difference depends upon whether the terminal event is anterior or posterior.

For the most part, this finding is without clinical significance as long as the QRS duration is less than .12 sec. The S_1 S_2 S_3 pattern has been attributed to a number of causes. The most frequent cause cited is the late activation of muscle tissue near the tricuspid or pulmonary valves. It is interesting to note that the terminal site of activation in the dog's heart is the base of the septum. This in itself could produce an S_1 S_2 S_3 configuration.

Distinction between an S_1 S_2 S_3 pattern and right bundle branch block is not always possible as both are associated with a terminal rightward vector. However, if congenital origin can be established, distinction is not important. If late activation of muscle tissue near the tricuspid or pulmonary valve is the cause, it is actually a delay in activation in the right ventricle.

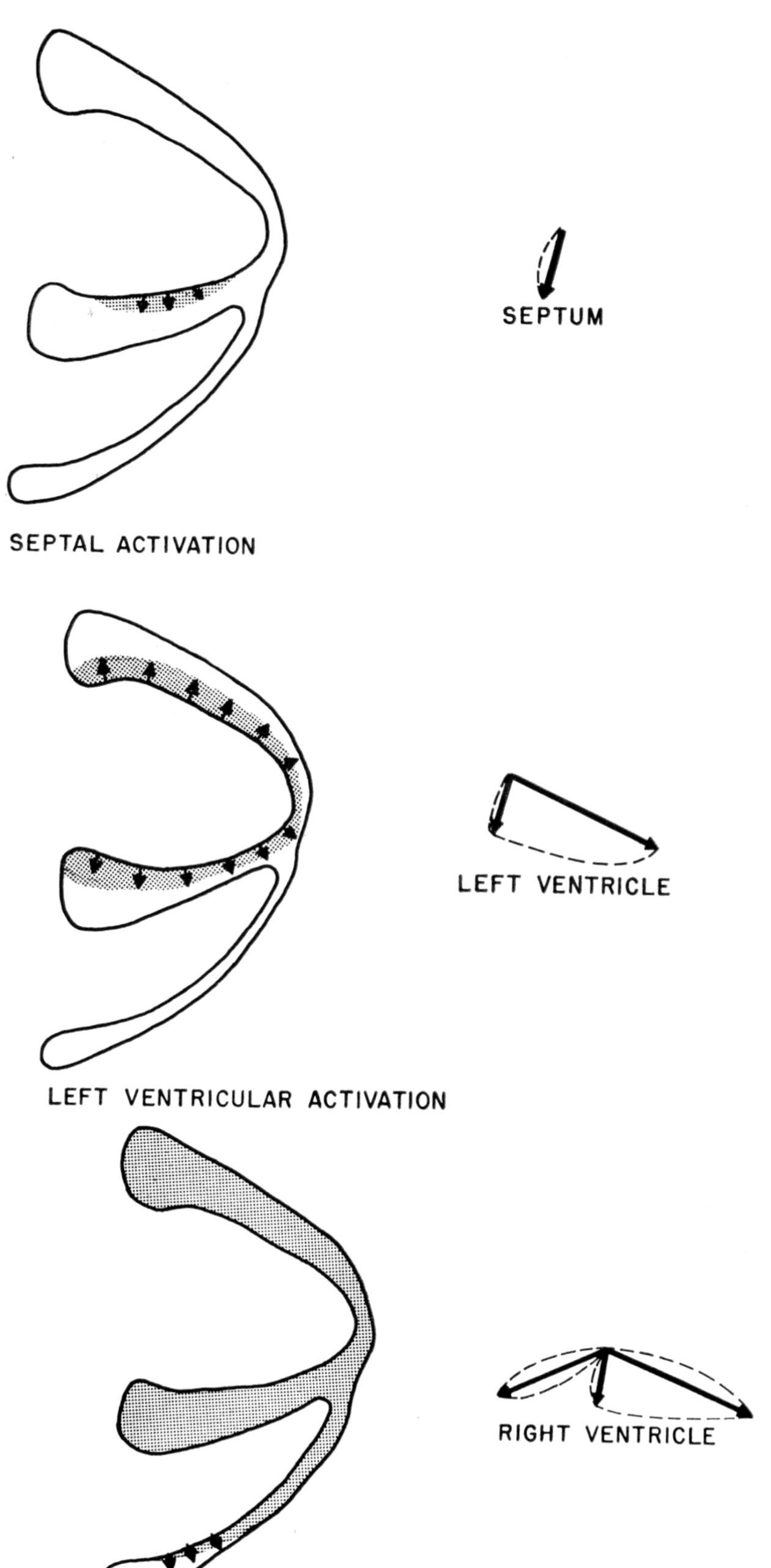

Figure 112. Order of ventricular excitation in right bundle branch block.

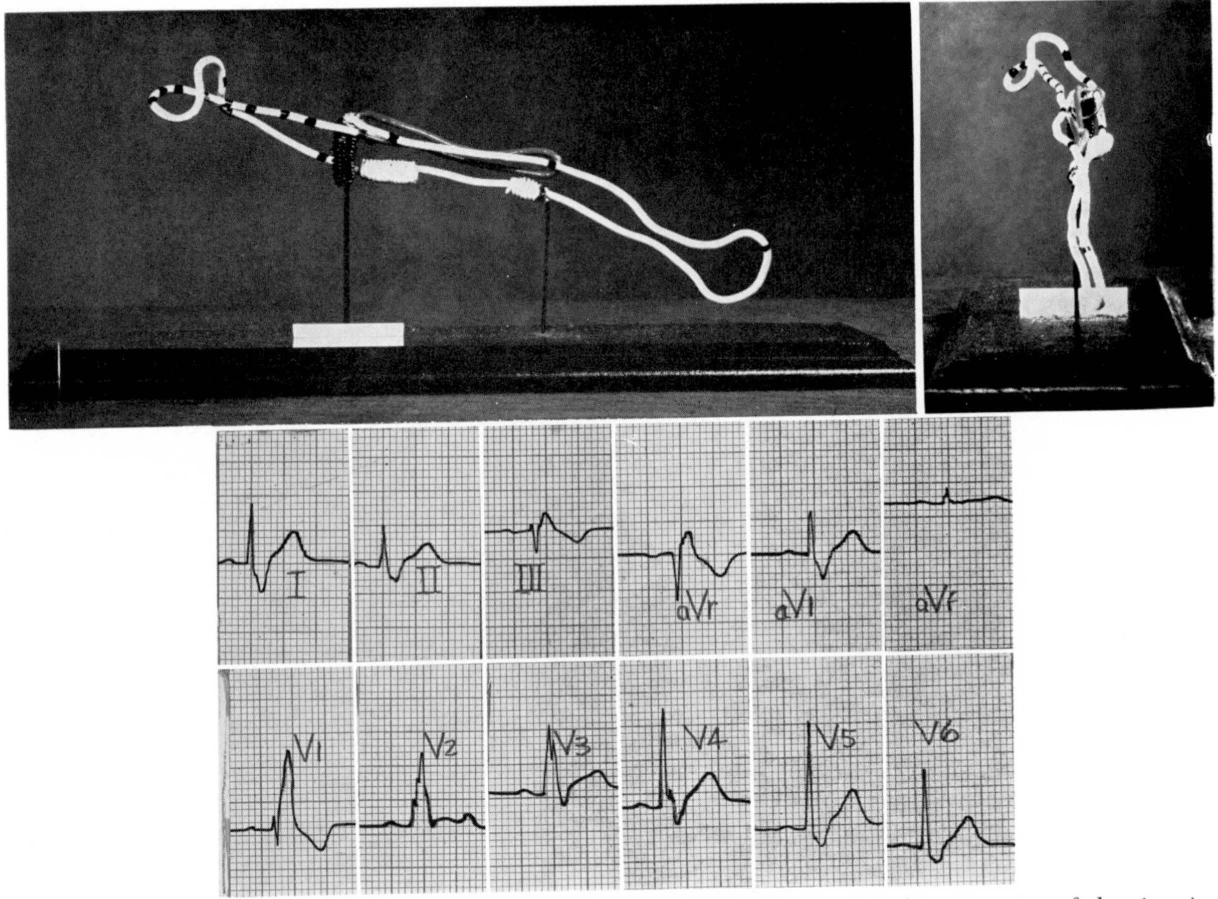

Figure 113. A twenty-five year old pilot with a right bundle branch block. The close grouping of the time intervals depicts the conduction defect.

INTRA VENTRICULAR CONDUCTION DEFECTS

A change in the order of excitation may occur at points other than the septum. The QRS configuration may be altered or the duration of excitation prolonged to nearly .12 sec. Occasionally these are called incomplete left or right bundle branch block. A better term is intraventricular conduction defect. The significance of this finding depends entirely upon its cause.

ACCELERATED CONDUCTION *(Wolff-Parkinson-White Syndrome, False Bundle Branch Block, Pre-Excitation)*

Normally there is a delay between the completion of atrial excitation and the onset of ventricular excitation. This delay is manifested by an isoelectric interval between the P wave and the QRS complex. In certain individuals ventricular excitation begins early or pre-excitation occurs. Often a localized muscle area is stimulated early and the remainder of the muscle is excited in the usual manner. This shortens the PR interval and prolongs the QRS duration. The classic form is a PR interval of 0.10 sec. or less and a QRS duration of .12 sec. or more (Figs. 117, 118, 119, 120, and 121).

Since the QRS duration is prolonged, it resembles bundle branch block. The clue is the short PR interval. Pre-excitation may occur in either the right or left ventricle and the QRS complex may resemble either right or left bundle branch block.

Two explanations have been advanced as cause for this finding. A bridge between the atria and the pre-excited area called the Bundle

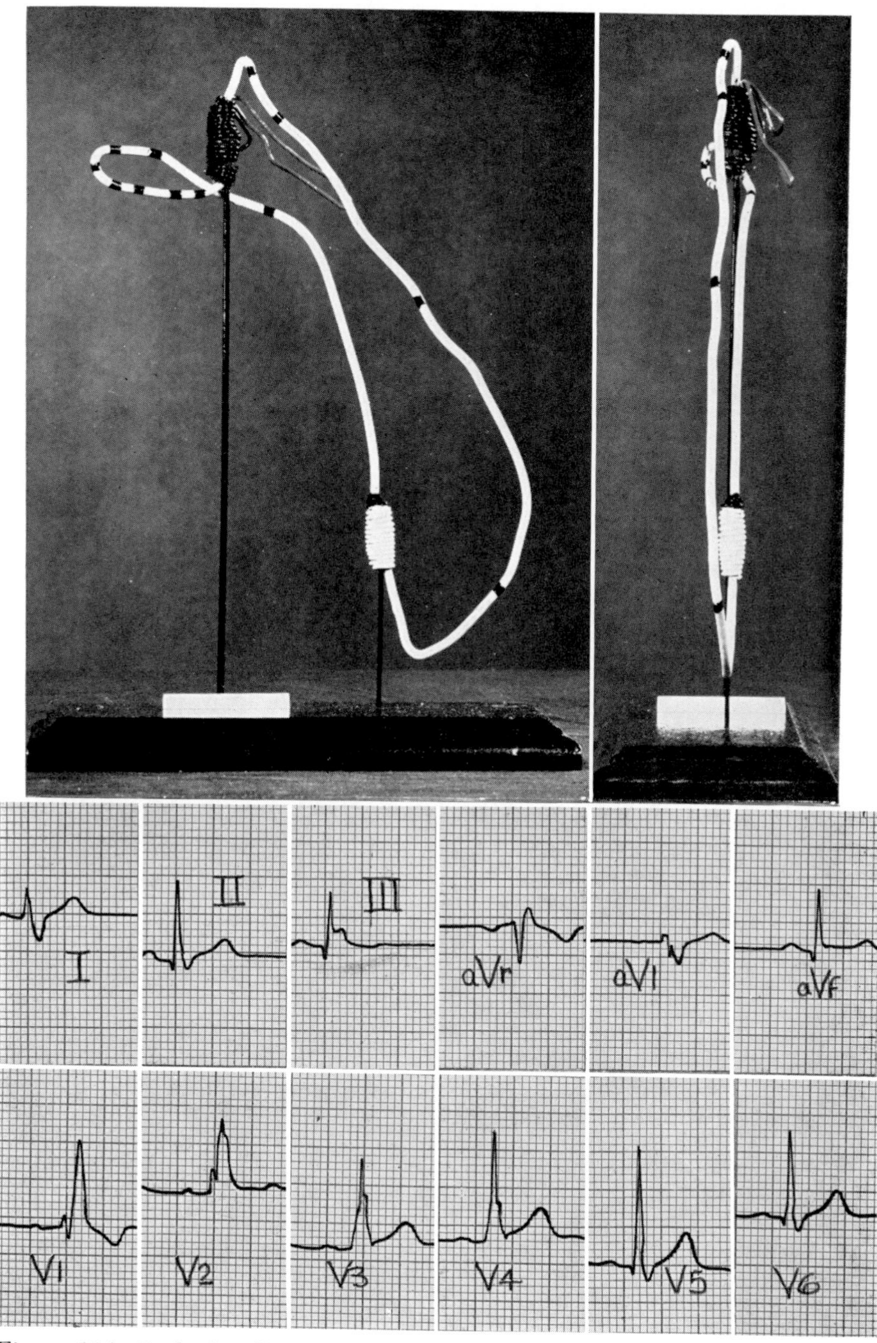

Figure 114. Right bundle branch block in an asymptomatic thirty-four year old physician.

of Kent was described as a means of early passage of the impulse around the AV node. Another explanation is to consider the AV conduction system as a central nervous system of the heart. An acceleration of conduction through one part of the node would stimulate its muscle receptor area early. This is called accelerated conduction. This has been demonstrated in the presence of nodal disease.

Regardless of the mechanism causing pre-excitation, it is clear that the excitation impulse must first pass over the atria to the region of the AV node, before pre-excitation can be set off, by accelerated conduction or through the Bundle of Kent. If the atria requires .12 sec. (normal value is .06 to .12 sec.) for activation, the pre-excitation phase must begin at .12 sec. or after a PR interval of .12 sec. In the event atrial excitation requires only .06 sec. a PR interval of .10 sec. gives a relatively normal period for delay between atrial and ventricular activation. The absence of a delay between completion of atrial excitation and the onset of ventricular excitation should be used to determine the presence of accelerated conduction rather than fixed values for the PR interval.

The muscle area undergoing pre-excitation creates a small force of slowly changing magnitude. This creates a slow early QRS pathway and on the ECG graph a slow onset of the QRS complex. The wave created by early onset is called the "delta" wave.

The T wave may be either normally directed or altered secondary to the change in the order of excitation. The accelerated cycles may not be constant, varying with respiration or alternating from cycle to cyle. Occasional normal records are recorded at intervals in the same subject.

Accelerated conduction is usually thought of as congenital in origin. However, accelerated conduction has been demonstrated in proved nodal disease. In hospital patients and those seeing a physician, 50 to 75% have recurrent paroxysmal tachycardia.

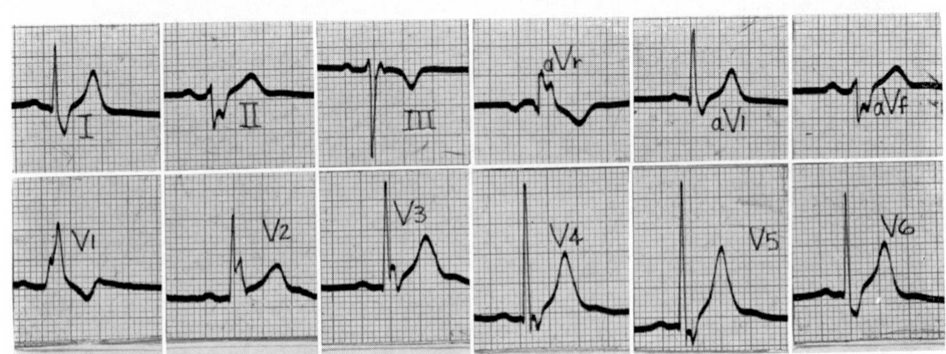

Figure 115. A thirty-four year old pilot's electrocardiogram of complete right bundle branch block. An electrocardiogram during childhood showed an intra ventricular conduction defect which remained unchanged until age twenty-two. At age twenty-six an electrocardiogram showed complete right bundle branch block which has remained unchanged for eight years. Catheterization studies were normal as were the remaining parts of the examination. It is of interest that he had coccidioidomycosis.

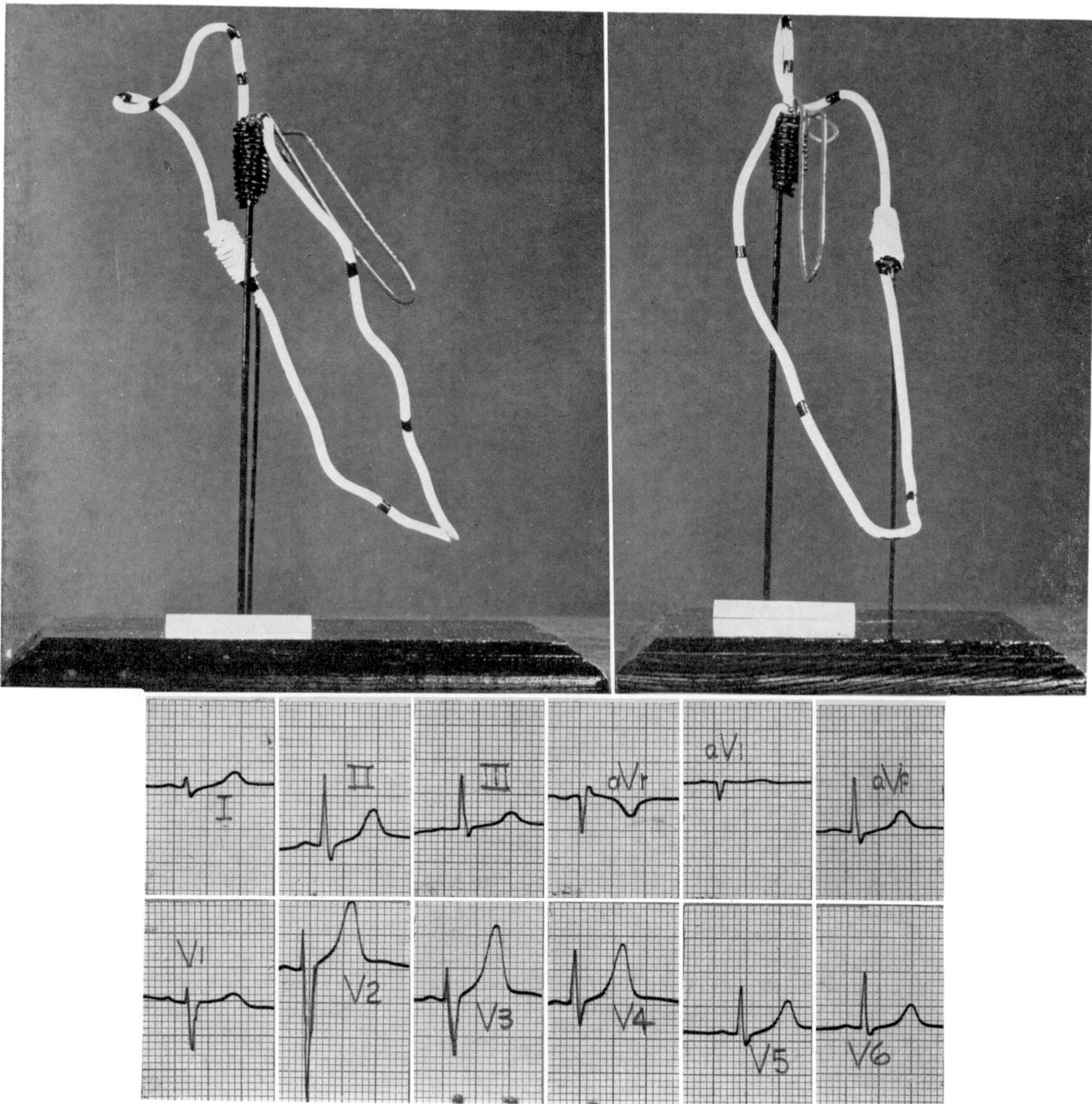

Figure 116. An S_1 S_2 S_3 pattern in a normal adult. The terminal QRS pathway is directed toward the right shoulder creating an S wave in Leads I, II and III. The close grouping of time intervals noted in right bundle branch block are not seen.

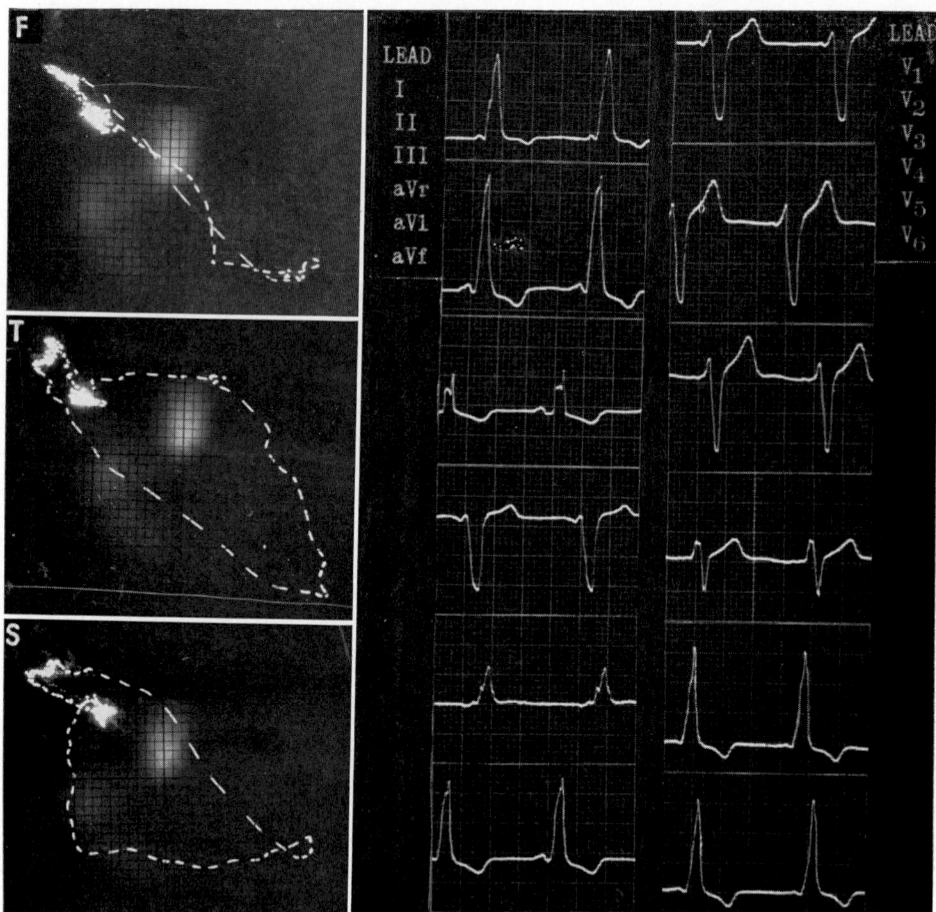

Figure 117. Accelerated nodal conduction in an asymptomatic twenty year old student. The short PR interval and prolonged QRS complex are characteristic. The prominent posterior course of the QRS pathway resembles left bundle branch block. The inverted T waves in Leads I, II and V6 are of no clinical significance.

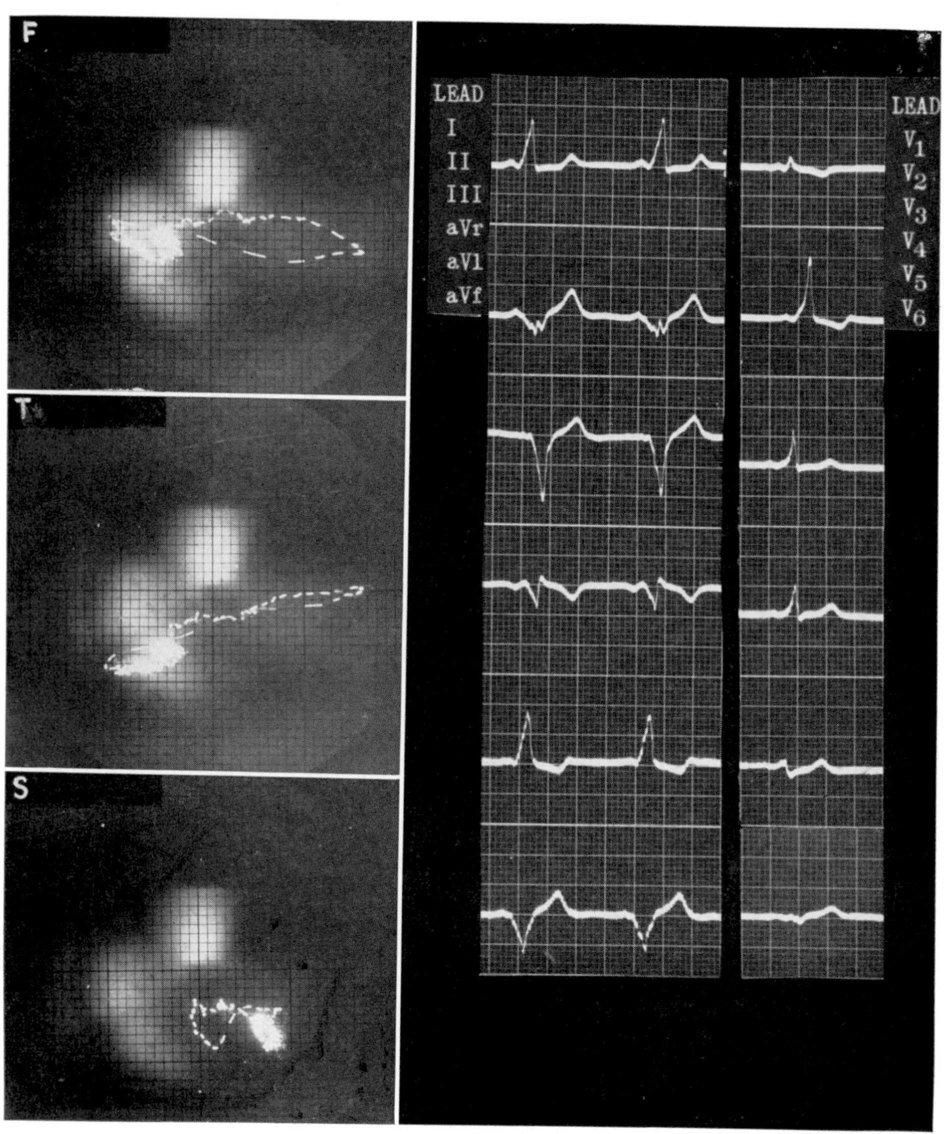

Figure 118. Accelerated nodal conduction in a forty year old woman. The slow conduction at the onset of the QRS is classical. The anterior orientation of the QRS pathway resembles right bundle branch block.

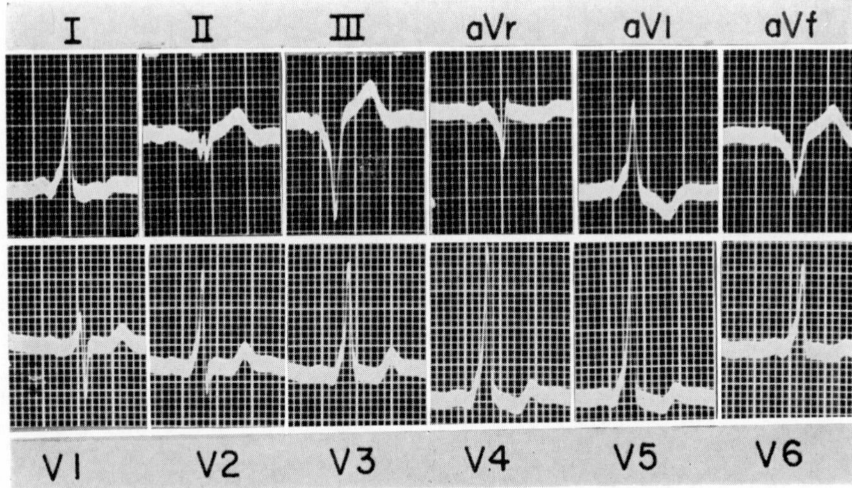

Figure 119. Accelerated nodal conduction in an eighteen year old boy found upon hospitalization for possible rheumatic fever. Subsequent investigation uncovered the same finding in records recorded during early childhood.

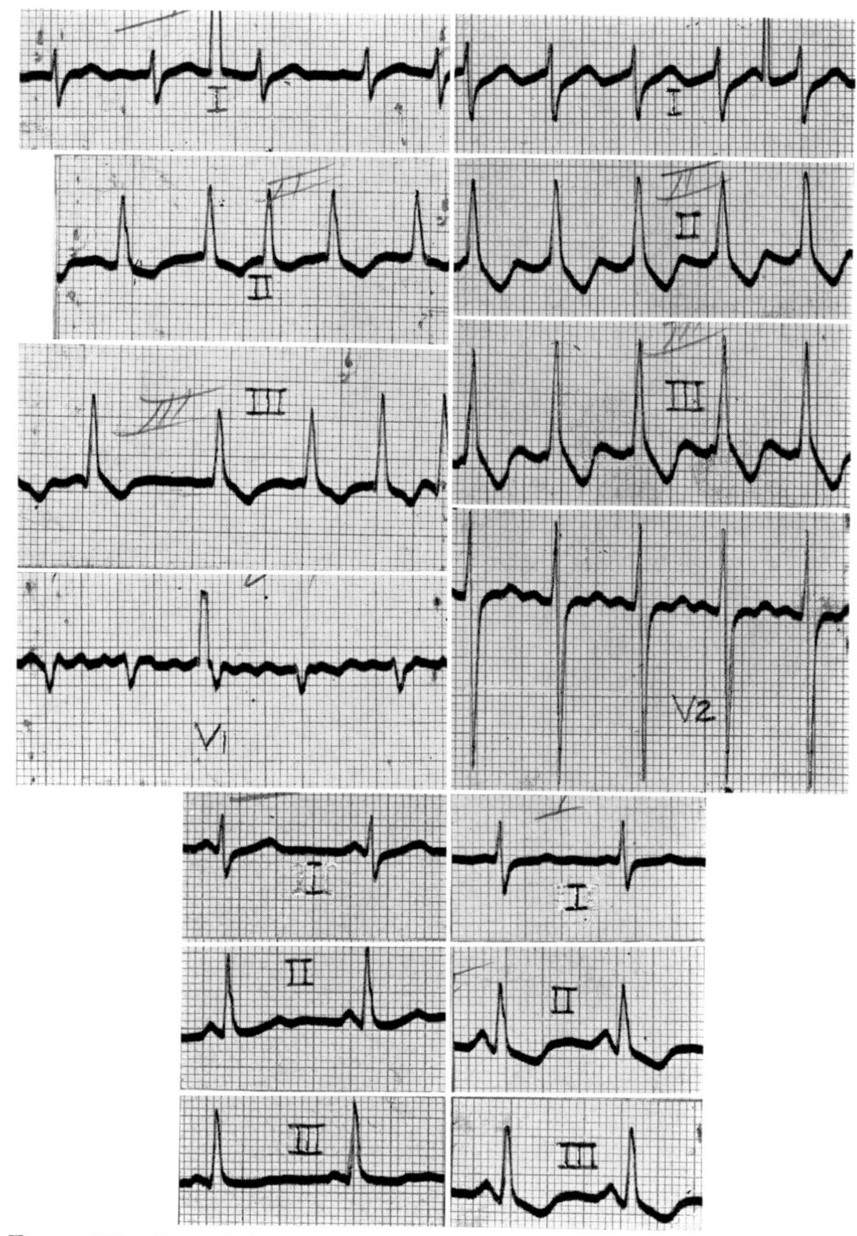

Figure 120. Upper left: On admission the patient had atrial fibrillation. Upper right: Sinus tachycardia (150/min). The small P wave runs into the QRS complex in Leads II and III. In V2 the sinus mechanism is readily apparent. Lower left: At normal rhythm the short PR interval of accelerated nodal conduction is seen. The QRS duration is within normal limits. Lower right: The P wave occupies .12 sec. causing the PR interval to be .12 sec. There is no isoelectric interval between the P wave and the QRS complex.

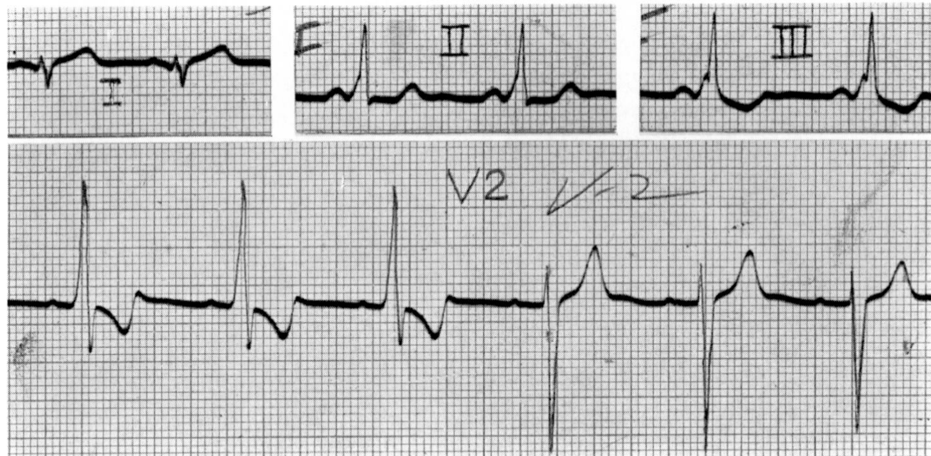

Figure 121. An example of accelerated nodal conduction that converts to normal conduction during recording of V2.

XI

Pericarditis

Acute pericarditis creates generalized epicardial injury. Injury current creates a force away from the zone of injury during the resting state and towards the zone of injury during the excited state. Thus the resultant vector of generalized epicardial injury is directed toward the base of the heart in the resting state and toward the apex in the excited state (Fig. 122).

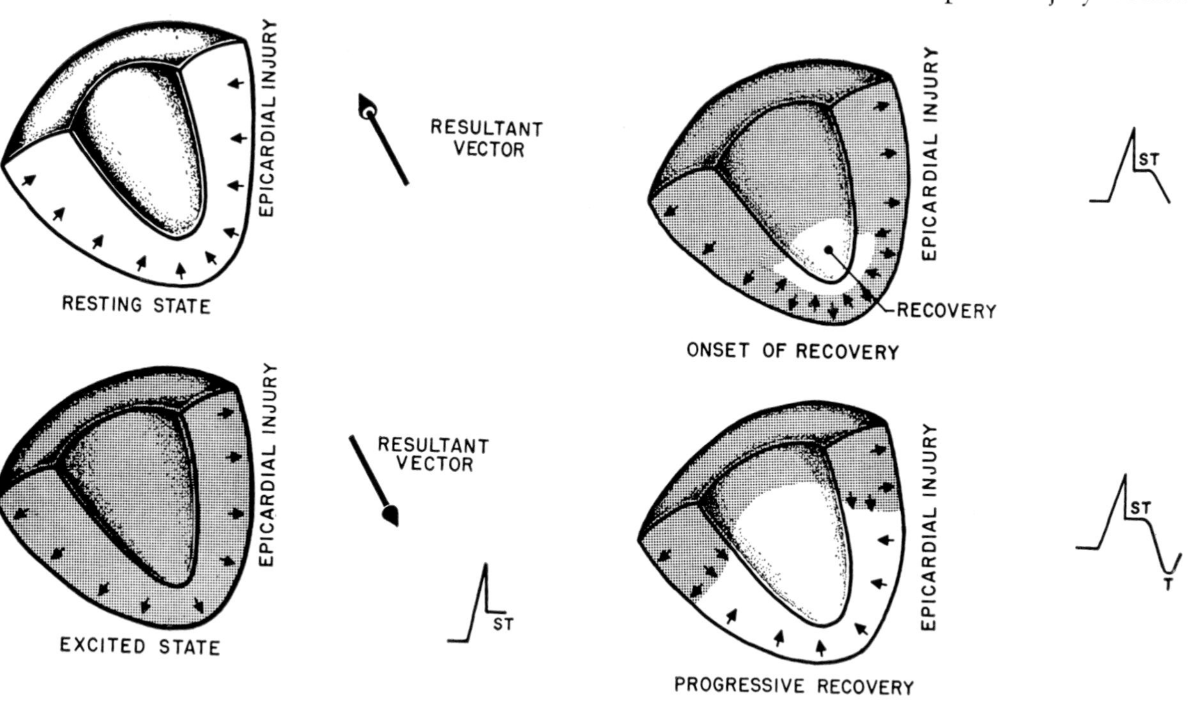

Figure 122.

The injury vector merely displaces the base line during the resting state so that the injury force is apparent only during the excited state. This is manifested by ST segment displacement. The apical direction of the vector in the excited state causes ST segment elevation in those leads with positive electrodes facing the heart and depression in leads with an electrode facing the base of the heart (aVr and Vl).

The injury vector during the excited state prevents the forces of excitation from returning to zero value (base line or point of origin) consequently the QRS loop remains open. The spatial vector directed from the point of origin to the ST interval is the spatial injury vector. Its length is proportional to twice the magnitude of resultant injury force.

Recovery proceeds normally from the endocardial surface. Its onset causes a decrease in the resultant injury force or a decrease in ST segment elevation. When the wave front of recovery reaches the surface the injury force is reversed towards the base of the heart (recovered tissue adjacent to injury has an injury force directed away from the area of injury). Thus the wave front of recovery forms a continuous shell with the epicardial region in the resting state. Effectively the wave front of recovery is an everted cone.

The force of recovery is opposite the force of excitation and is manifested by an inverted T wave following an upright QRS complex or a T loop opposite the QRS loop. The T vector is commonly small when the injury vector is large. As the injury vector diminishes in magnitude, the T vector magnitude increases. The elevation of an ST segment in leads with an inverted T wave has given rise to the rule that *abnormal ST segment deviations are present when the ST vector is directed opposite the T vector whereas normal ST segment displacement occurs with the ST vector and T vector directed in the same direction* (Fig. 123). Serial records provide the best evaluation of the significance of ST segment displacement.

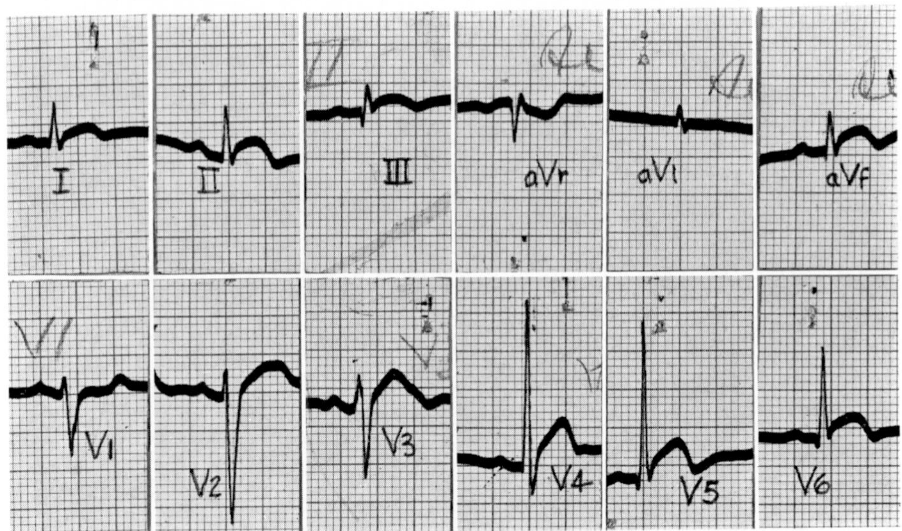

Figure 123. ST segment and T wave changes of acute pericarditis.

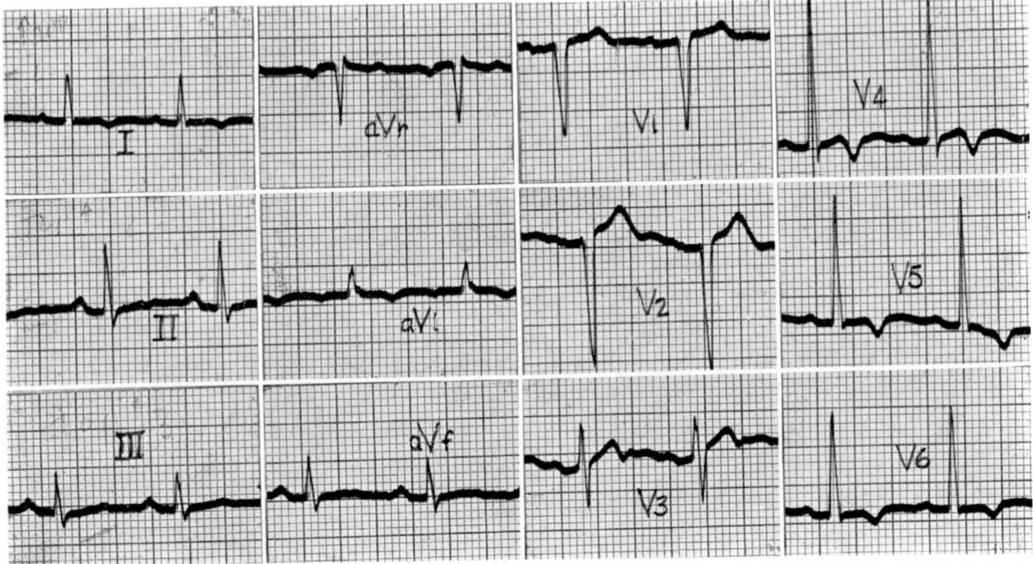

Figure 124. Chronic pericarditis with permanent T wave changes.

As the area of injury subsides, the magnitude of the injury vector diminishes. This results in closure of the QRS loop, or return to normal of the ST segments. With complete healing of the injured area, new cell membranes are formed and no constant current exists. T wave inversion may persist for an indefinite period of time following acute pericarditis and in some instances is permanent (Fig. 124). The scarified tissue over the myocardium creates local tension by pulling on the subjacent muscle tissue. Such mechanical action causes abnormal delay in epicardial recovery. Consequently, the wave front assumes the shape of an everted cone with forces directed towards the base of the heart.

Pericarditis may be associated with decreased QRS amplitude. This may be caused by: 1) actual muscle damage by inflammation or calcium deposits, with diminished density of change on the wave front, 2) increased heart rate in the febrile state, or 3) cardiac compression diminishing cardiac volume and the size of the wave front, either by effusion or constriction. Pericardial effusion occurs in the acute stage. Constriction occurs in the chronic form of pericarditis.

XII

Myocardial Infarction and Arteriosclerotic Heart Disease

MYOCARDIAL INFARCTION

INFARCTION OF THE MYOCARDIUM results from deficient blood supply to a muscle area. This may be due to increased need or decreased supply or a combination of the two. The most common cause of myocardial infarction is arteriosclerotic heart disease with coronary artery thrombosis. Coronary artery thrombosis is not entirely analogous to experimental ligation of the coronary artery, because coronary thrombosis most often occurs in an individual with diseased arteries. The disease is not necessarily confined to the thrombosed vessel.

The myocardium receives its blood supply from the right and left coronary arteries. The arteries arise from the base of the aorta and extend over the ventricular surface. The right coronary artery and its ramifications extend over the posterior surface. The left coronary artery extends over the anterior and posterior ventricular surface. Ramifications of these arteries extend inward through the myocardial wall. The smaller vessels extending from the larger vessels create an interlacing network at the endocardial shell.

A number of conflicting viewpoints have been presented by various authorities to explain the ECG findings of infarction. To cite one major incompatibility, consider the concept that infarction involves chiefly the endocardial surface. If this is true, the laws of injury current are incorrect. The forces of injury are directed toward the zone of injury during the excited state, therefore a large endocardial infarction zone would create an ST force away from the zone of infarction (Fig. 125).

The factual information based on empirical observations is as follows:

1) Infarction may occur without any significant changes in the routine ECG.

2) Infarction may be manifested only by T wave changes in the routine ECG (Fig. 126).

3) The classical ECG pattern in infarction

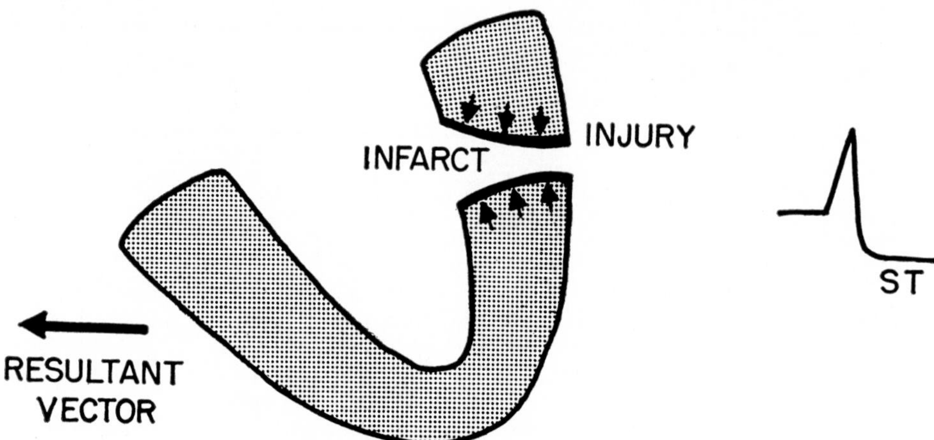

Figure 125. When endocardial infarction is larger than the epicardial region the ST vector is directed away from the site of injury rather than toward the infarction.

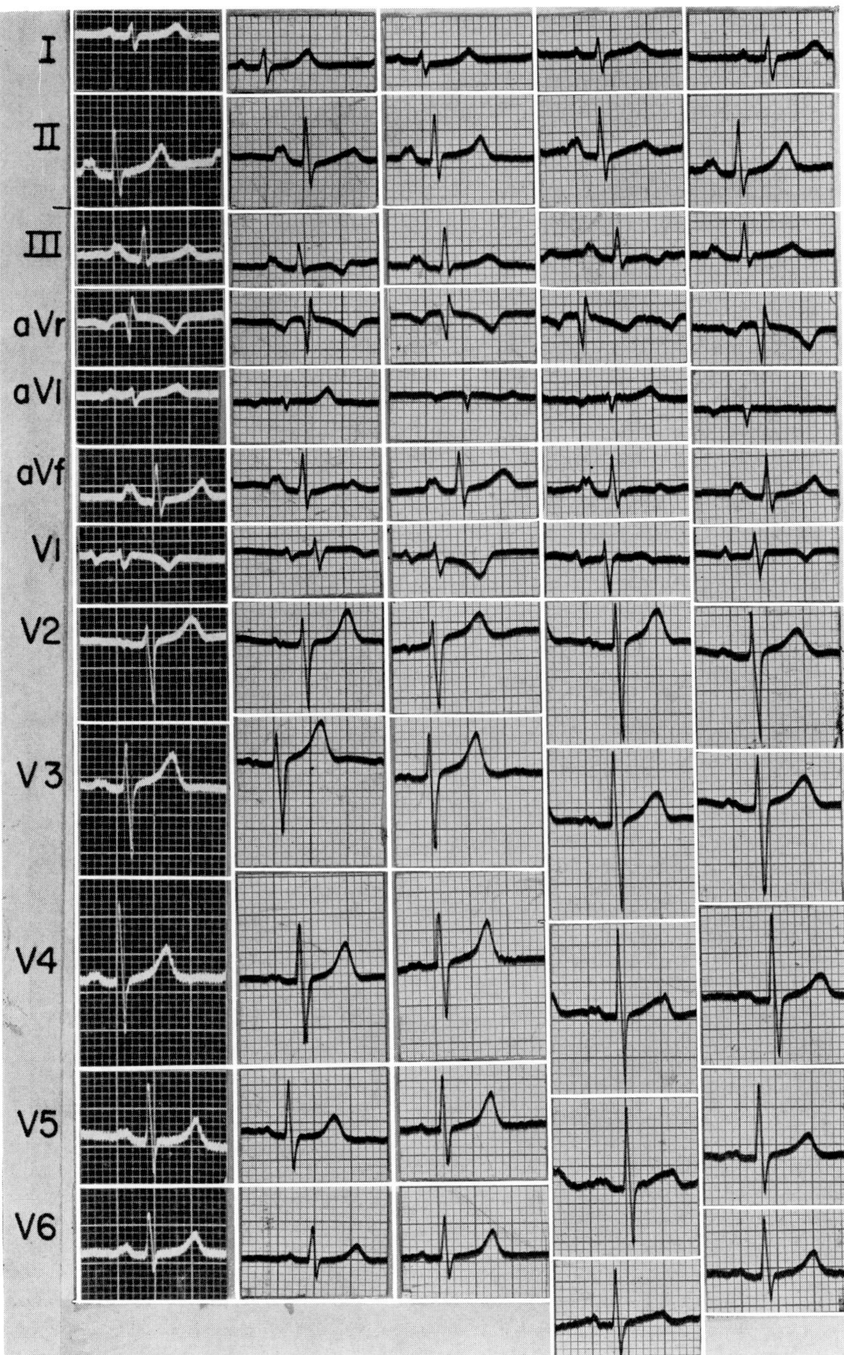

Figure 126. A) Base line ECG six months before illness in a fifty-seven year old man. B) Approximately 18 hours after minor chest discomfort. The only significant change is the T wave in Lead III. C) Three weeks later the T wave has gradually returned to its upright position. There are minimal ST segment changes in Leads I, II and V1 (not sufficient for a definitive diagnosis alone). D) Four weeks later following an episode of syncope while having his hair cut. At four weeks and three days the electrocardiogram showed its maximum changes, of minor T wave changes. He had clinical infarction pain and laboratory findings following the episode of syncope. E) Seven weeks from onset the ECG appeared almost identical to the base line record. At eleven weeks he died suddenly without warning. Autopsy findings demonstrated diffuse scarring of the anterior wall of the left ventricle with long standing disease of the anterior coronary artery. The septum showed diffuse scarring of healed injury. There was thrombosis of the right coronary artery.

consists of an initial Q wave of .04 sec. duration, an elevated ST segment and an inverted T wave in those leads with a positive electrode facing the infarcted area. This is a changing pattern with gradual return toward normal and in some instances complete return to normal.

4) T wave changes persist in a portion of records and abnormal Q waves persist in others.

5) Infarction may present an initial finding of very large T waves that are upright, rather than the classic inversion described above (Fig. 127).

6) Infarction may decrease the QRS amplitude or the length of the QRS pathway.

7) Discrepancies in the location of the infarction at post-mortem examination and the location indicated by the ECG can be attributed in part to eccentric zero center location and variation in lead lengths.

Bayley's* classic experiments on ligation of the coronary artery have often been used as an explanation of the sequence of infarction. In considering the experimental findings it is well to remember that coronary artery disease was not present and presumably normal coronary flow occurred through the rest of the arterial tree.

The earliest change noted after ligation was inversion of the T wave. T wave changes were followed by ST segment elevation. If the vessel was tied a sufficient length of time, a Q wave appeared.

It seems logical that if one considers the endocardial shell relatively deficient in blood supply it would be the first area to suffer from hypoxia under these circumstances. This would result in a larger upright T wave, not an inversion. Injury should affect the endocardial shell first and this would produce an ST segment depression. On the other hand, if the epicardial shell is relatively deficient in blood supply, the T wave and ST segment changes observed are compatible with the basic concepts of hypoxia and injury. The endocardial shell normally re-

*Bayley, R. H., and LaDue, Electrocardiographic changes of impending infarction and ischemia injury pattern produced in the dog by total and sub-total occlusion of a coronary artery. *Am. Heart J.*, 28:94, 1944.

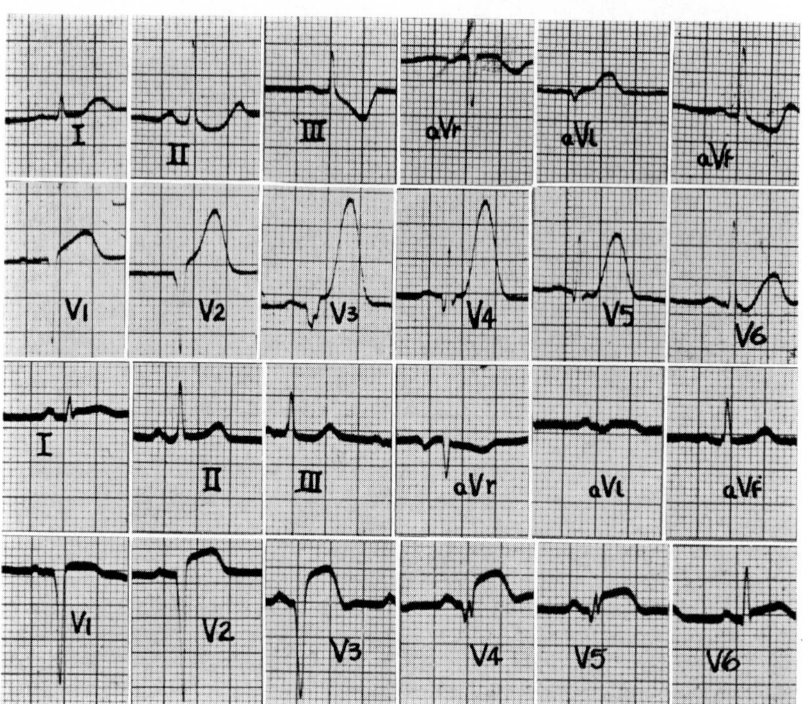

Figure 127. An example of large upright T waves at the onset of anterior infarction (above), and inverted precordial T waves in subsequent records (below).

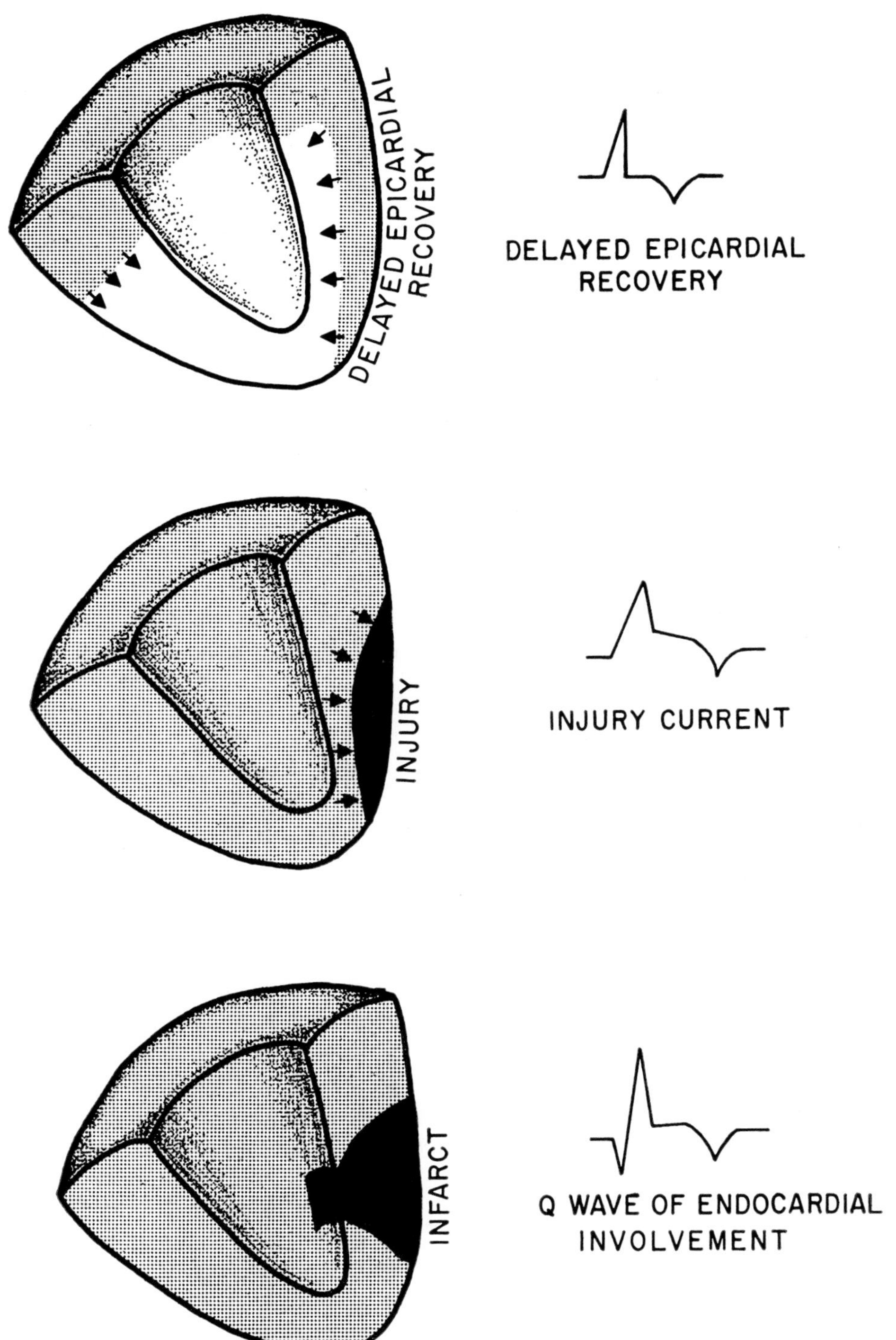
DELAYED EPICARDIAL RECOVERY
DELAYED EPICARDIAL
RECOVERY
INJURY
INJURY CURRENT
INFARCT
Q WAVE OF ENDOCARDIAL
INVOLVEMENT
EXTENSION OF INFARCTION
TO ENDOCARDIAL SHELL

Figure 128.

ceives some blood supply from both major vessels. This probably accounts for the earlier changes in the epicardial region. If hypoxia persists, the entire thickness of the myocardial wall becomes infarcted. Involvement of the endocardial shell creates the abnormal Q wave (Fig. 128).

A comparable situation occurs in the patient with localized coronary artery disease and thrombosis. Early T wave changes are followed by ST segment elevation and abnormal Q waves. The classic infarction may be defined in vector terminology as follows:

1) An initial .04 QRS vector directed away from the area of infarction.

2) An ST vector directed toward the area of infarction.

3) A T vector directed away from the area of infarction.

Using these rules, infarctions may be classified as to location. There are four principal locations: anterior, posterior, lateral, and diaphragmatic. Combinations of these areas may be involved (Figs. 129, 130 and 131).

The initial forces of excitation are directed away from the infarcted area by the hole the infarction makes in the wave front. This will be the dominant effect of a transmyocardial infarction until the conical wave fronts begin to change, i.e., the completion of right ventricular

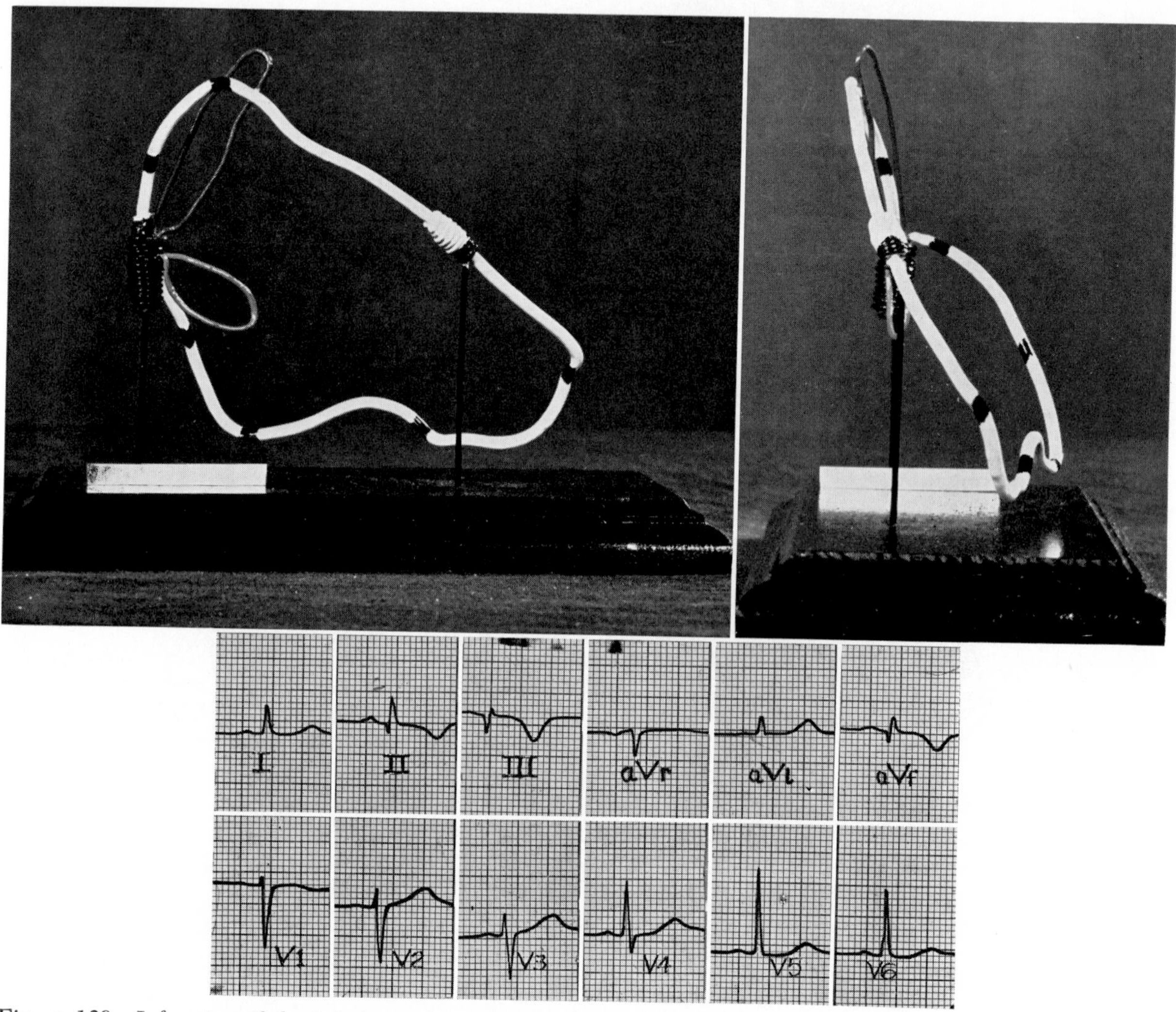

Figure 129. Infarction of the inferior surface of the left ventricle creates an upward initial course of the spatial QRS pathway. The T loop is directed away from the area of infarction. This is depicted by the Q wave and inverted T wave in Leads II, III, and aVf. The size of the QRS loop is small.

and septal activation. This period of time roughly corresponds to .04 sec. This has given rise to the clinical observation that infarction creates abnormal Q waves with a duration of .04 sec. Depending upon the location and size of the infarct, the remainder of the QRS pathway may be increased or decreased in size. After the wave front has passed the level of infarction the QRS pathway assumes its normal course and magnitude.

Characteristic QRS changes are the most reliable hallmark of infarction. ST and T waves are important, but they are not always good indicators of the location of the infarction, and may be due to many other causes.

The early, large, upright T waves may be explained on the basis of transmyocardial hypoxia. In the event of shock or disease of other coronary vessels the endocardial shell will not enjoy the additional blood supply from collateral cir-

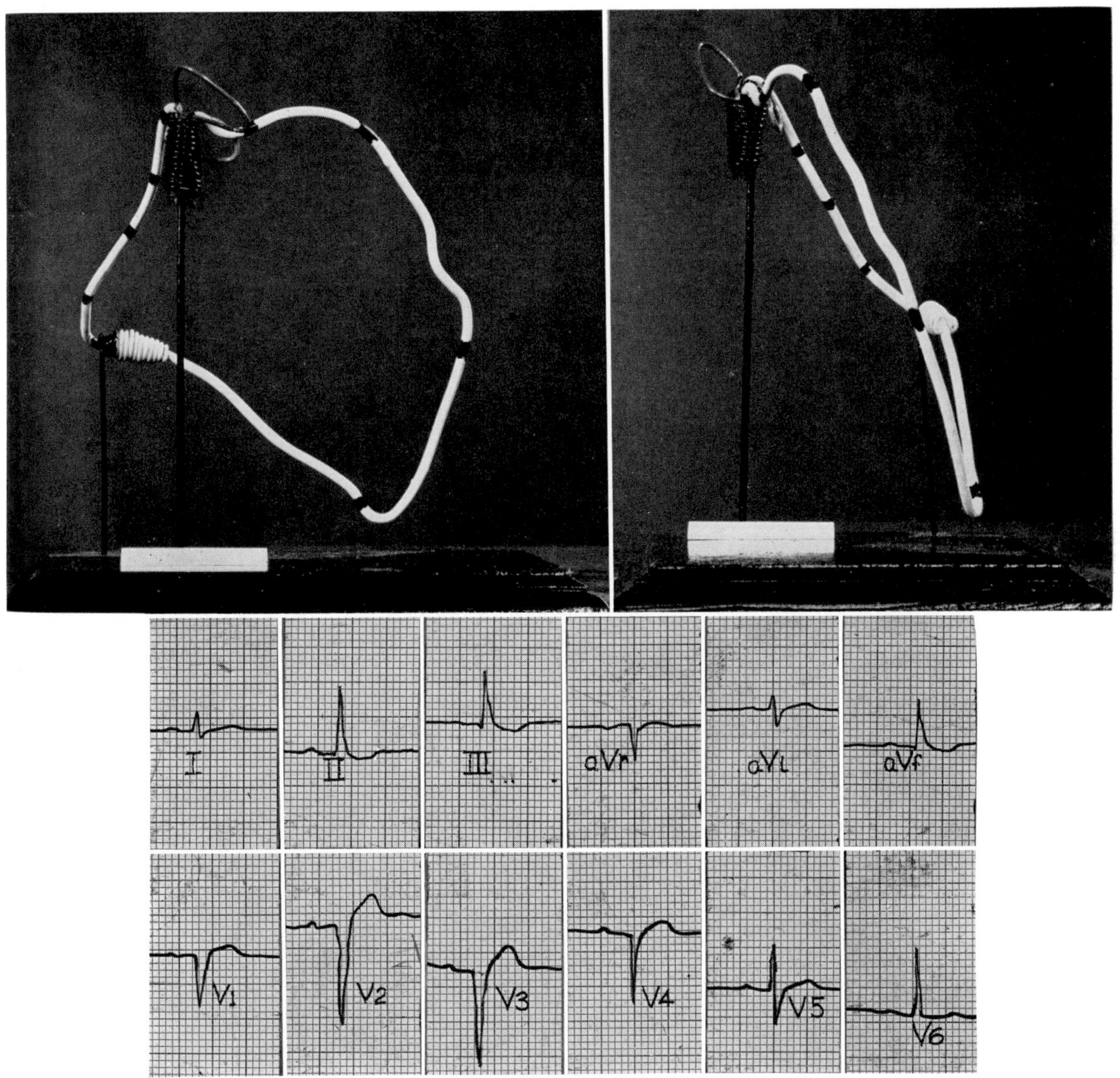

Figure 130. An example of anterior wall infarction. The QRS loop is directed entirely posterior. This is represented by QS deflections in V1, V2, V3 and V4. The QRS loop is small. This individual's first evidence of infarction occurred eleven years ago.

culation. Occlusion of a vessel will cause an immediate hypoxia of the entire wall thickness followed quickly by injury and necrosis.

Diffuse endocardial infarction is deserving of special comment. Infarction of the entire endocardial shell will be apparent only as an ST injury force directed toward the base of the heart. There is no hole in the wave front of excitation. A complete infarction of the entire endocardial shell without extension through the myocardial wall is rather rare (Fig. 132).

The problem of endocardial infarction also concerns the depth of infarction. Infarction extending only 3 millimeters into the wall will occupy a time interval of only .01 sec. This time interval is so short it may not be recorded by the usual direct writing instrument.

In order to alter the initial process of excita-

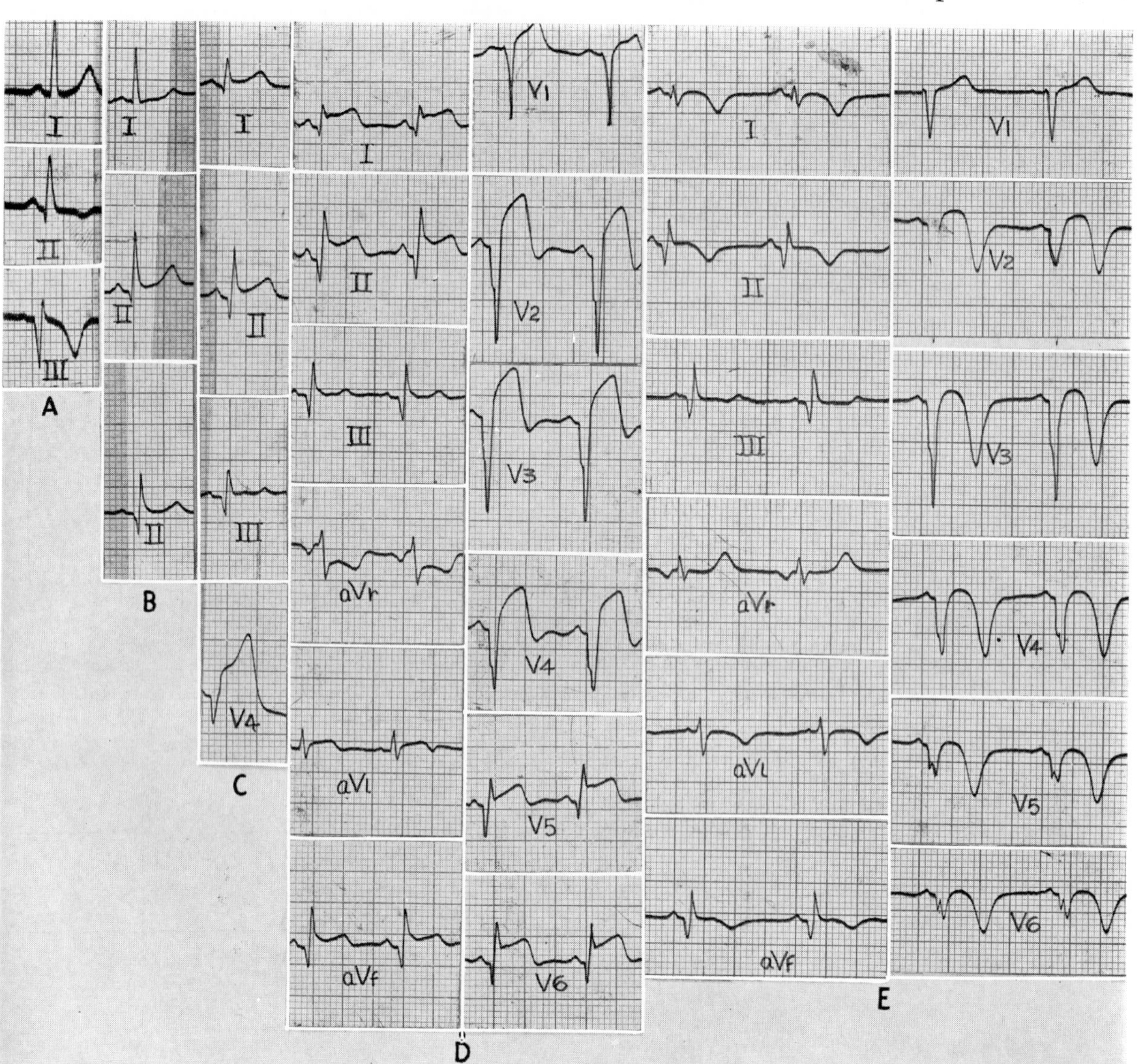

Figure 131. A) Electrocardiogram in 1947, five days after chest pain, showing inferior wall infarction (Q_3T_3). B) In 1952 the Q wave in Leads II and III persisted but were smaller. C) One week later, two hours after moving furniture, Lead I and V4 show a new infarction. D) The following morning a typical acute anterior wall infarction, superimposed upon an old inferior wall infarction is evident. E) Two weeks later the acute elevation of the ST segments has subsided and there are deep inverted T waves in Lead I and V2 through V6. The area involved is the anterior lateral surface of the left ventricle. Note the loss of QRS amplitude in Lead I with the loss of the muscle area responsible for the leftward force of excitation.

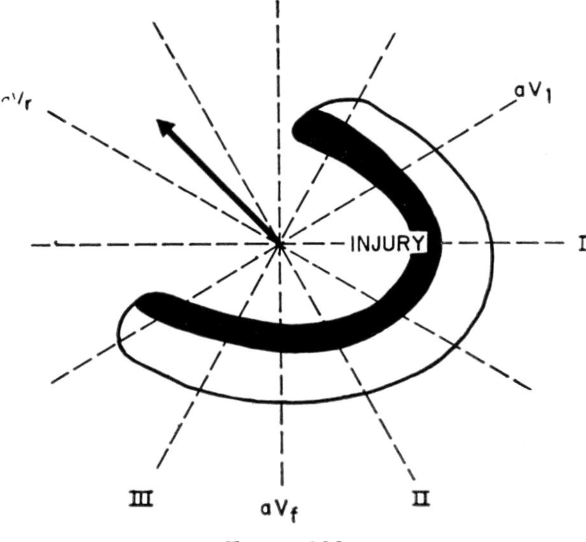

Figure 132.

tion, infarction must involve the endocardial shell. The duration of the influence of infarction depends upon the distance the infarction extends outward. The magnitude of the change in force depends upon the area of infarction. A small infarction, creating a small hole in the wave front, will not appreciably alter the direction of the resultant force of excitation.

The wave front of excitation for the left ventricle normally represents a cone at .02 sec. Its resultant force is perpendicular to the base of the cone, or the base of the left ventricle. An infarction (hole) in the cone will tend to rotate the resultant. The new resultant force may be depicted as the resultant from the conical base area and the infarction area (Fig. 133). The larger the hole, the greater is its effect on rotation of the resultant. One cannot expect the manifested forces during excitation to point directly away from the anatomic site of infarction unless the area of infarction is quite large.

Diffuse or patchy muscle necrosis creates no appreciable change in the direction of the forces. A localized area of necrosis within the wall thickness extending neither to the endocardial or epicardial surface will cause changes only midway in the excitation cycle. This is one cause for QRS notching.

Infarction involving only a portion of the outer myocardial shell will not be manifested

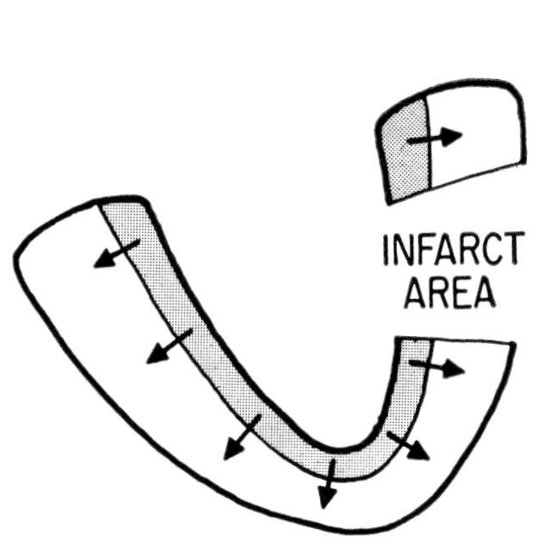

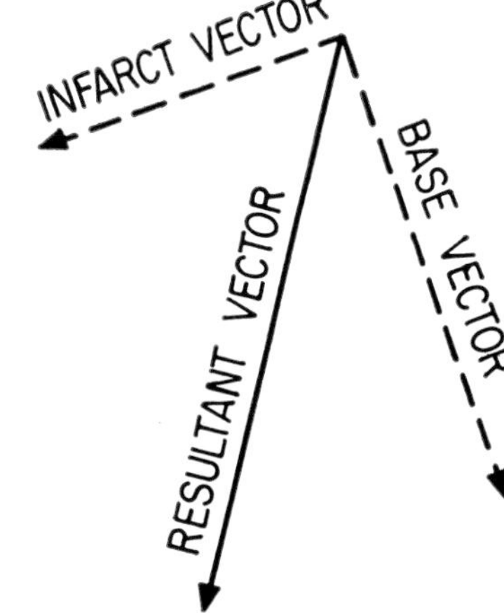

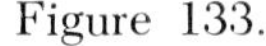
Figure 133.

in the early portion of the excitation cycle. It will influence magnitude and direction of the later events of the cycle. Considering the above relationships, it is not surprising that infarctions may be manifested only by ST segment and T wave changes when studied by a routine ECG. While the ECG is a very valuable diagnostic adjunct in myocardial infarction, it does not replace the clinical diagnosis. Serial electrocardiograms demonstrating serial changes in conjunction with the clinical picture remains the most satisfactory approach at this time.

ARTERIOSCLEROTIC HEART DISEASE

Diffuse coronary artery disease causes changes in cellular metabolism. Diffuse fibrosis may occur. With loss of normally functioning cell mass there is a decrease in ion density across the wave front of excitation. This can cause decreased QRS amplitude. The vectorcardiogram in terms of electrical moment clearly depicts the change (Fig. 129). A low QRS voltage after infarction favors generalized myocardial disease.

An occasional finding in arteriosclerotic heart disease is ST segment depression followed by an upright T wave. This has been explained as due to endocardial hypoxia. This finding is accentuated with exercise, or during acute coronary pain. During an anginal attack there may be transitory T wave inversion. Acute ST segment depressions should always be respected as a possible indication of endocardial injury and impending infarction. Serial records should be obtained.

Arteriosclerotic heart disease may cause left axis and widening of the mean spatial QRS-T angle. The T vector may be rotated more leftward than zero degrees. The QT interval may be prolonged.

At present the diagnosis of arteriosclerotic heart disease by the ECG in the absence of infarction or acute changes with angina is difficult and the tracing may appear normal. However, magnitude measurements have never been refined and measurements in terms of electrical moment should improve the diagnostic technique.

XIII

Drugs and Metabolism

DIGITALIS

Digitalis affects the basic electrical events of the cardiac muscle fiber. It alters the membrane action potential during the recovery phase. This phase is associated with an increased outward migration of potassium ions. Digitalis increases the permeability of the cell membrane to potassium ions, accelerating the outward potassium current. Clinically, digitalis is given to increase the strength of muscular contraction. The refractory and contractile response of muscle fibers is closely related to intracellular potassium content. The effects on the recovery phase increase with increasing concentration of digitalis. At toxic levels the early period of the membrane action potential is altered, diminishing the initial spike. Since the early events of the membrane action potential are associated with an increased inward migration of sodium ions, the permeability of the membrane to sodium ions must be altered at these concentrations.

At theraupeutic levels digitalis increases the speed of recovery of the ventricles. With more rapid spread of endocardial recovery the wave front assumes the form of a large inverted cone. This produces a force toward the base of the heart during the ST interval (excited state). A normally directed resultant vector toward the apex is created when the wave front reaches the epicardial surface (Fig. 134). This vector is diminished in size and duration due to the extensive early recovery of the endocardial shell. The larger the endocardial shell of recovery prior to recovery of the external surface, the larger will be the ST force and the smaller the recovery (T) force. The enhancement of endocardial recovery produced by digitalis has three principal effects:

1) Shortening of the QT interval.

2) Creation of a vector (ST) during the excited state in the opposite direction of the excitation (QRS) vector, and opposite the normal recovery vector (T).

3) The larger the ST interval vector, the

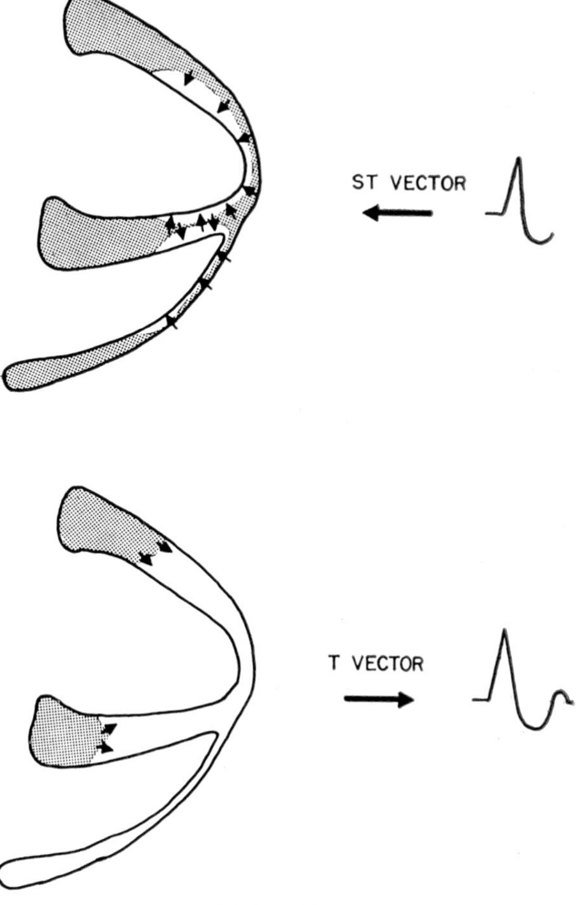

Figure 134.

smaller the T vector. It is apparent that complete recovery throughout the endocardial shell will result in a short QT interval with a large ST force and little or no apparent T force (Fig. 135).

The ECG findings of digitalis effect do not indicate intoxication, nor can they be used as a reliable index for the proper dosage of digitalis.

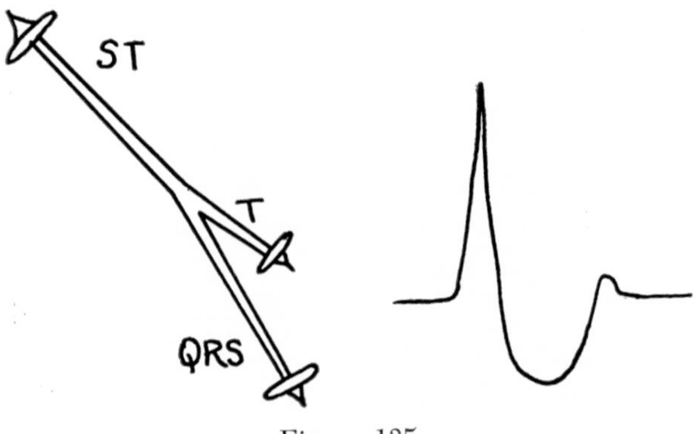

Figure 135.

In toxic doses, extra systoles may occur (Fig. 136). Digitalis can cause multiple forms of arrhythmias. In toxic doses it may increase the PR interval but toxicity may occur before the PR interval is significantly prolonged. When the T vector has been previously altered due to other causes, e.g., left ventricular hypertrophy, the chief effect is shortening of the QT interval and change in character of the ST segment (Fig. 137).

QUINIDINE

Quinidine causes prolongation of all the electrical events of the heart. The QRS complex and QT interval are both prolonged by administration of quinidine. Most likely quinidine acts by altering the capability of the cell membrane to transmit excitation and recovery impulses. The direct action on the cell membrane decreases the threshold of irritability. This action enables quinidine to be effective in the treatment of arrhythmias.

By slowing the outward transmission of recovery along the cell membrane, endocardial recovery will create a force during the excited state (ST segment) before the apparent stage of recovery (T wave). The ST segment change is similar to that seen in left ventricular hypertrophy. Quinidine may slow recovery to the extent it creates a large persistent everted cone, inverting the T waves. Danger of cardiac standstill from quinidine is real if the ECG is not used to detect increasing QRS duration when large doses are used. With increasing concentration of quinidine, transmission of impulses is progressively slowed. The main ECG features of quinidine are:

1) Prolongation of PR interval.
2) Increase in P wave size and duration.
3) Increased QRS duration.
4) ST segment depression.
5) QT interval prolongation.
6) T wave may become inverted.

HYPOPOTASSEMIA

When the concentration of potassium ions in the extracellular fluid decreases, there is an increased outward migration of potassium ions during the recovery phase. Recovery is closely related to the outward current of potassium ions. Apparently when the intracellular and extracellular potassium ion concentration ratio reaches a critical level the membrane recovers. With extracellular hypopotassemia a larger quantity of intracellular ions must migrate outward to create the critical ratio. The prolongation of the recovery phase enables the creation of wave fronts or currents within the endocardial shell. This is reflected in the ECG by ST segment changes.

The characteristic ECG findings in hypopotassemia are:

1) Prolongation of the QT interval.
2) ST segment deviations.
3) Diminished amplitude of the T wave (Fig. 138).

If hypopotassemia persists, the constant increased outward migration of intracellular potassium ions results in cellular potassium depletion. Since the contractility and excitability of the cell is directly related to potassium ion

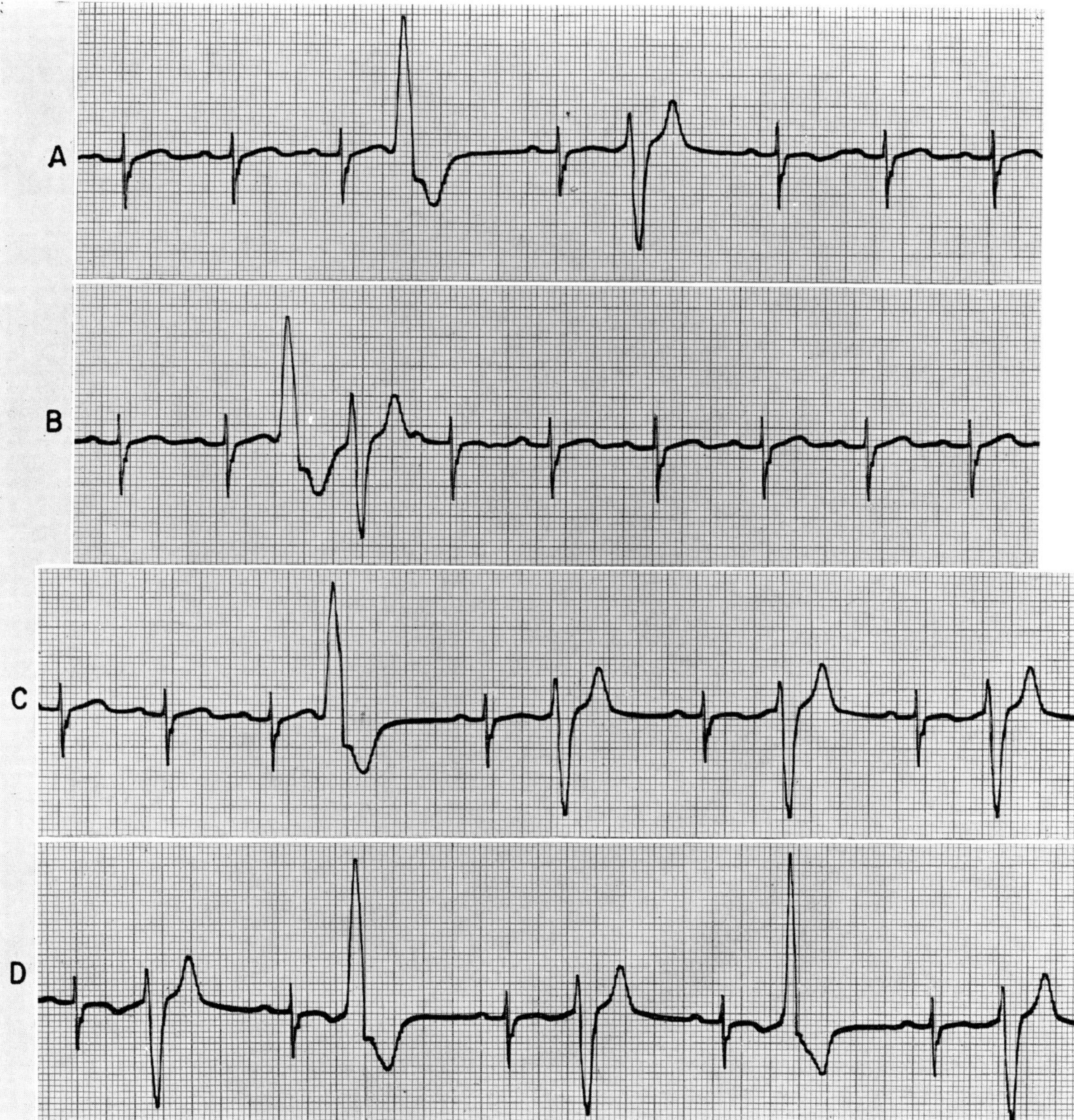

Figure 136. Digitalis intoxication. A) Ventricular premature contractions occurring from two foci. B) Coupling of impulses from the two foci. This may occur when the second focus initiates an impulse during the supernormal phase of excitability of the ventricle. C) The onset of bigeminy due to a ventricular prematurity every other beat. D) Alternating bidirectional bigeminy with the two foci alternating in creating ventricular premature contractions. All these rhythms occurred in a short time interval in one patient.

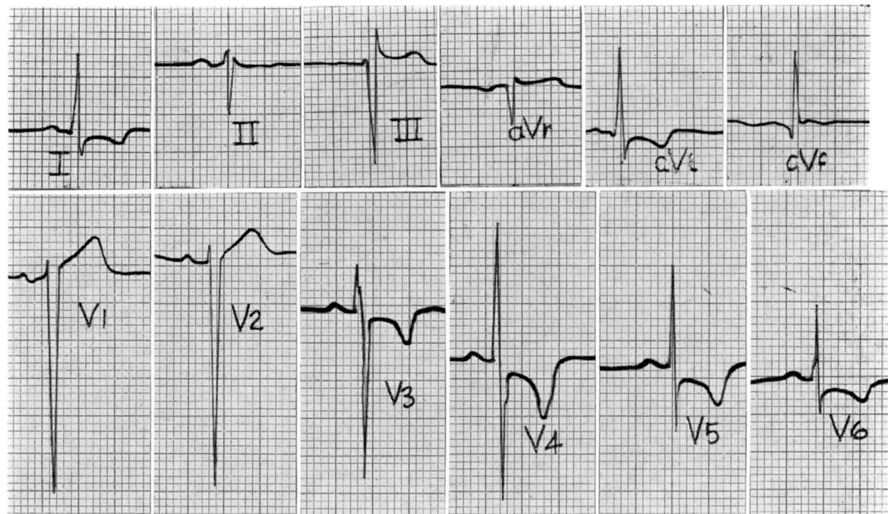

Figure 137. The same patient as seen in Fig. 103 after digitalization. The QT interval is shortened from its previous duration.

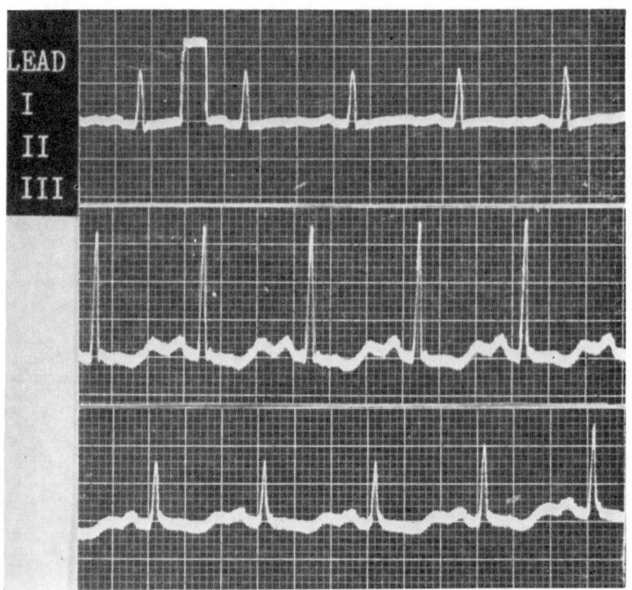

Figure 138. Prolongation of the QT interval and ST segment depression due to hypopotassemia.

concentration, it is not surprising that arrhythmias occur.

Digitalis intoxication and hypopotassemia both create intracellular potassium ion depletion.

HYPERPOTASSEMIA

Elevation of the extracellular potassium ion concentration shortens the recovery stage. A smaller amount of outward potassium ions migration is required to reach the critical intracellular/extracellular ratio. Recovery is rapidly transmitted to the epicardial surface, increasing the demonstrable force of ventricular recovery. The shortening of the recovery period (ST interval) with increased force results in the tall peaked T waves of hyperpotassemia.

As the extracellular level of potassium ion concentration increases, the outward driving force for potassium ion migration, created by the difference in intracellular and extracellular ion concentration, diminishes. When this force is effectively abolished, standstill occurs. The atrium is first affected. P waves disappear due to atrial standstill. At progressively higher extracellular concentrations, ventricular response is altered. Excitation becomes more difficult and the QRS complex widens. Fusion of the QRS and T waves occurs resulting in a scrambled electrocardiogram of biphasic waves. The distinction of excitation and recovery is not possible. Ventricular standstill is the final phase of hyperpotassemia.

CALCIUM

Very little is known about the action of calcium ions in excitation and recovery. Diminished calcium ion concentration results in delay of the onset of recovery. This is manifested by prolongation of the QT interval with no apparent changes in character of the ST segment or T wave. Increased calcium ion concentration shortens the QT interval and may increase T wave amplitude or cause rounding of the T wave. Calcium has a synergistic action with digitalis.

THYROXIN

Thyrotoxicosis causes increased cardiac output. This is accomplished by increased heart rate with an increased or normal stroke volume. The ECG shows tachycardia and normal or increased QRS amplitude. Myxedema causes decreased cardiac output with diminished stroke volume and bradycardia. The ECG shows a slow heart rate and diminished QRS amplitude. The QRS amplitude may reflect either change in cell function with deposition of extracellular material in the heart or decreased stroke volume. Pericarditis with effusion may be an accompanying feature.

XIV

Arrhythmias

SINUS RHYTHMS

Normal Sinus Rhythm. The SA node, atrium, AV node and ventricular endocardium are all under the influence of vagal inhibition and sympathetic acceleration. The SA node controls the cardiac rate and is called the pacemaker. In infants the normal rate may be between 100 and 150. The normal rate decreases with advancing age and in the adult the normal rate is 60 to 100.

When the impulse from the atrium reaches the AV node, there is a delay before ventricular excitation. This allows sufficient time for atrial systole prior to ventricular systole. In normal sinus rhythm the length of time for the impulse to pass from the SA node to the ventricle is dependent upon the length of time for the impulse to pass over the atria and the period of transmission through the AV conduction system. The normal adult PR interval is never less than .10 sec. and never more than .21 sec. In large adults with a cardiac rate below 70, the PR interval may be .21 sec. The method of exact measurement of the PR interval is discussed earlier in the text (Fig. 139).

Sinus Tachycardia. The impulse originates in the SA node and traverses the rest of the cardia in normal fashion. The rate in the adult is over 100 per minute. Sinus tachycardia may be defined as a sinus rate above the normal rate for that particular individual. Sinus tachycardia is usually not thought to exceed a cardiac rate of 160 per minute. Rare instances of rates above that level have been noted. The onset of sinus tachycardia is insidious and its termination is gradual. The cardiac rate varies from minute to minute. Carotid sinus pressure causes perceptible smooth slowing of the cardiac rate. This is transient in nature and the original rate returns during pressure. Performing this maneuver during the recording of the tracing is absolutely essential in establishing the diagnosis (Fig. 140).

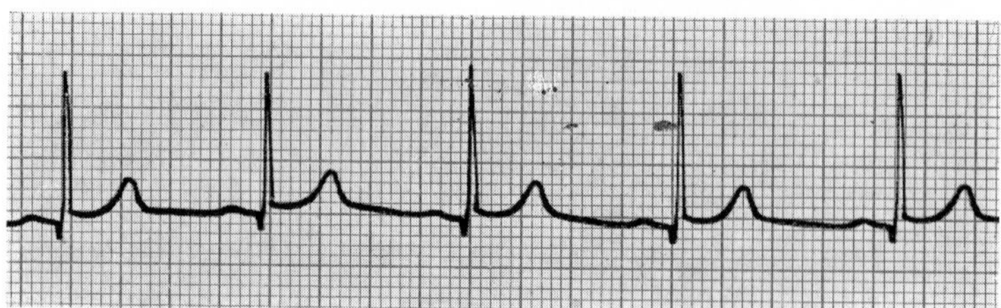

Figure 139. Normal sinus rhythm, rate 75 per minute.

Sinus tachycardia is occasionally associated with aberrant conduction. This permits an abnormal order of ventricular excitation resulting in abnormal QRS complexes.

Sinus tachycardia is due to changes in nervous regulation, myocardial function, or increased venous return. With mild exertion the pulse rate increases 20 to 40 beats per minute but falls to normal limits within two minutes. When treatment is necessary, the first step is to correct the underlying cause, e.g., hyperthyroidism, if such is present, or replacement of blood in the face of acute blood loss.

Sinus Bradycardia. When a sinus mechanism is present at a rate of less than 60 per minute it is a sinus bradycardia. This may be a normal finding in young athletes. It has been reported present in individuals without demonstrable heart disease at rates as slow as 33 per minute. Sinus bradycardia with mild cardiac enlargement may be a normal finding and be merely

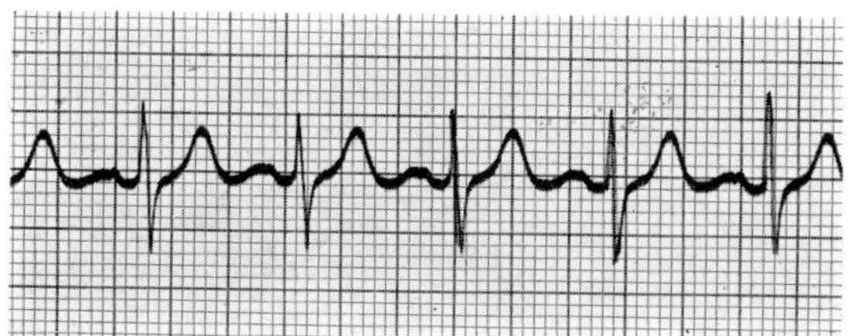

Figure 140. Sinus tachycardia, rate 110 per minute.

an "athlete's heart" with cardiac dilatation due to increased stroke volume.

Sinus bradycardia is commonly seen in central nervous system involvement and certain infectious diseases, including hepatitis. A relative bradycardia is seen in typhoid fever.

Sinus bradycardia is usually asymptomatic. Occasionally individuals will experience dizziness or syncope. It may be a manifestation of a sensitive carotid sinus and when associated with symptoms this reflex should be tested by massage of the carotid sinus during the time the ECG is recorded (Fig. 141).

Sinus Arrhythmia. Sinus arrhythmia is the cyclic change in rate associated with respiration. The rate increases at the onset of inspiration and slows at the height of inspiration or at the beginning of expiration. When this arrhythmia presents confusion in diagnosis, having the patient hold his breath during the recording will disclose the nature of the disorder.

Vagal inhibition of the cardiac rate is at a minimum at the onset of inspiration (cross effect of the Herring Brewer reflex). Increased venous return to the right heart occurs with inspiration due to negative intrathoracic pressure and the increased capacity of the pulmonary vascular bed.

When the breath is held in full inspiration there is often marked slowing of the heart rate. This reflex slowing may be more evident than carotid sinus slowing. I have observed momentary cardiac arrest and AV block from holding the breath in full inspiration.

Sinus arrhythmia is common in the young, but it is also common in the elderly and the arteriosclerotic. It requires no treatment (Fig. 142).

Sinus Arrest. In sinus arrest no impulse originates from the SA node and consequently the entire cardiac cycle is lost. The cycle which is lost may not equal a full length cycle. Sinus arrest cannot be clinically distinguished from sinoauricular block in which no impulse is transmitted from the SA node despite stimulation. If sinus arrest persists for several cycles without another rhythm occurring, it is cardiac arrest and constitutes a cardiac emergency. Sinus arrest is usually precipitated by vagotonia and may be one manifestation of a hypersensitive carotid sinus (Fig. 143).

ATRIAL RHYTHM

Atrial Premature Contractions. Whenever the electrical events of the heart are initiated

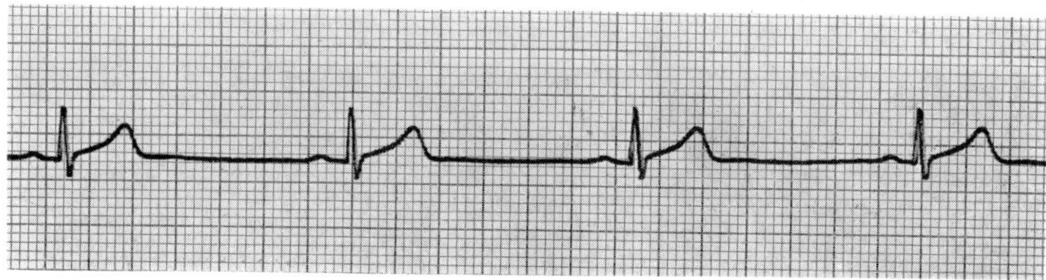

Figure 141. Sinus bradycardia, rate 45 per minute.

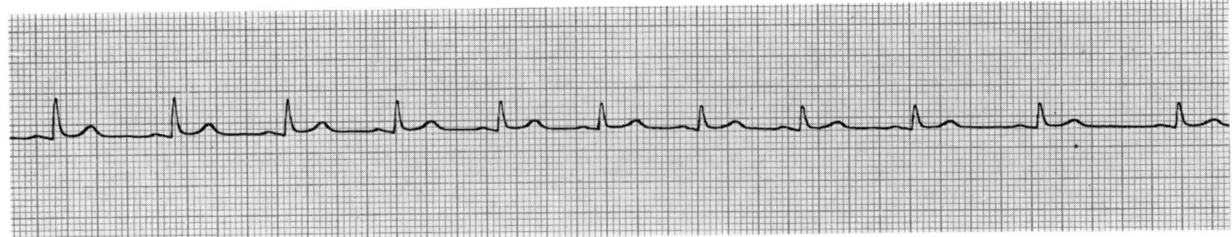

Figure 142. Sinus arrhythmia, rate approximately 80 per minute.

prematurely by a focus within the atria it is called an atrial premature contraction. The normal sequence of excitation does not occur and the P vector is altered. The PR interval may be entirely normal if the focus is far removed from the AV node. If the focus is close to the AV node, the PR interval may become shortened.

The QRS complex is usually like those of normally conducted beats, being associated with normal excitation. Less commonly early ventricular excitation occurs near the focus causing an abnormal QRS complex. This has been called aberrant conduction.

Usually there is a longer pause after the prematurity than the usual TP interval. This pause is not so long as to make a complete compensation for two successive cycles. This lack of compensatory pause is the chief method of establishing the diagnosis at the bedside. The pause is not compensatory because the atrial impulse causes the SA node to discharge, thereby interrupting its normal rhythmic discharge. Whenever a prematurity from any focus fails to interrupt the normal rhythmic discharge of the SA node and the node discharges during the prematurity, the pause is completely compensatory.

When atrial premature contractions are noted in a patient with a history of paroxysmal rapid heart action, it is a clue that the disorder is atrial tachycardia.

Atrial premature contractions: 1) occur prematurely, 2) are followed by a pause that is not completely compensatory, 3) have a normal or shortened or even prolonged PR interval, 4) have a normal or abnormally directed P vector, and 5) commonly have a normal QRS complex (Fig. 144).

Atrial Tachycardia. An atrial premature contraction may initiate an attack of rapid heart action with an atrial focus as the pacemaker. This is atrial tachycardia. The rate is regular and is usually between 150 and 250 beats per minute. In infants it may be as rapid as 300 beats per minute.

The onset of the attack is sudden and it ends just as suddenly. A sudden motion may precipitate such an episode. The rate will not vary more than two beats per minute. When the episode is terminated there may be a fairly long

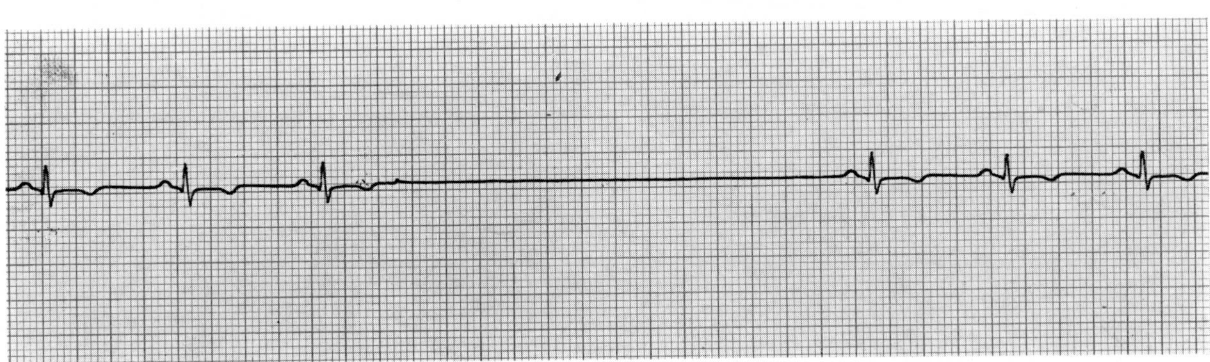

Figure 143. Sinus arrest.

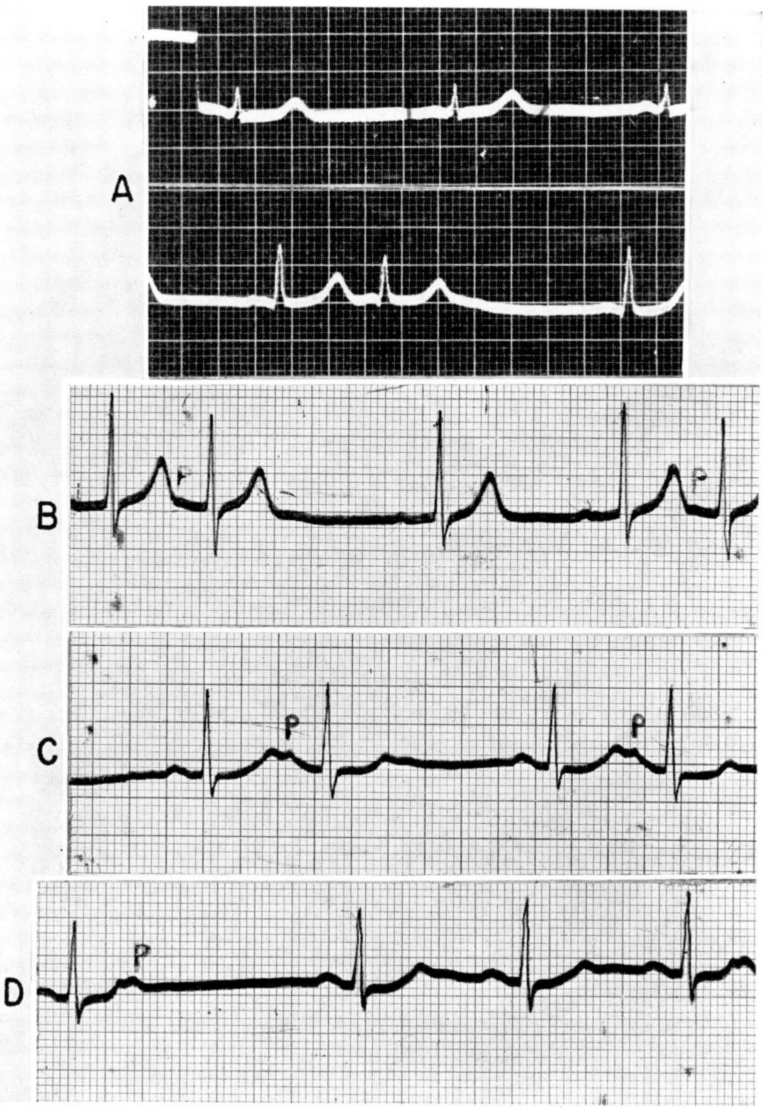

Figure 144. A) Normal rhythm above and prematurity occurring below. B) Two atrial premature contractions. C) Prematurities creating coupled rhythm. D) A blocked atrial premature contraction.

pause. Rarely has cardiac arrest occurred when the attack stopped. Short paroxysms of ventricular tachycardia have been said to occur at the time of termination.

Carotid sinus stimulation never affects the rate unless it stops the attack. This maneuver is not always successful and is of benefit in perhaps as few as 50% of the cases. Other manipulations to increase vagotonia may be used, including eyeball pressure and gagging (Fig. 145).

Atrial Flutter. As the atria become more irritable they respond more rapidly to a single focus and their rate is increased. When atrial response to stimulation is as rapid as 200 to 360 per minute it is atrial flutter. The exact mechanism of atrial flutter is not known. It may be initiated with one focus or by multiple irritable foci. The electrocardiographic findings are the same and consist of a rapid atrial rate, a P vector directed in the axis of 90°, and usually a regular ventricular response.

Only part of the atrial impulses are transmitted to the ventricle but this is commonly at a regular rate, e.g., every other impulse transmitted, or one in six impulses transmitted. The regular transmittal rate results in a regular ventricular response. If the atria are responding at a rate of 300 per minute and every other impulse is transmitted, the ventricles will contract 150 times per minute. This is called a two to one flutter. If only one in four impulses were transmitted the ventricular rate would be 75 per minute and this would be a four to one flutter. Ventricular response is not always regular, and the flutter rate may vary between a three to one and a four to one rate. Many different combinations may exist. The regular atrial rate between 200 and 360 per minute with a regular ventricular response usually presents no difficulties in recognition (Fig. 146).

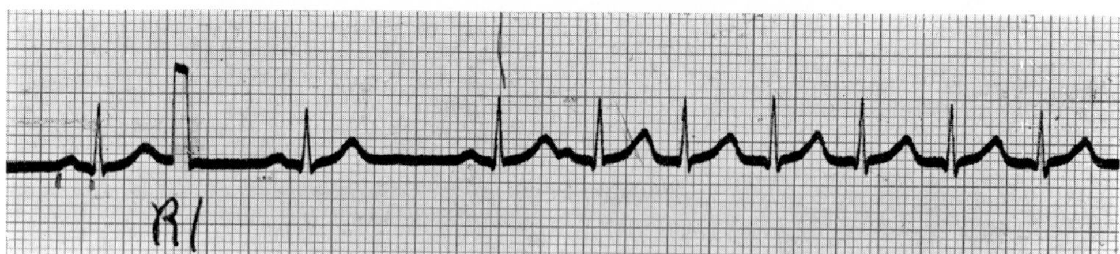

Figure 145. Paroxysmal atrial tachycardia.

Atrial Fibrillation. When atrial excitation is as frequent as 350 to 500 per minute atrial fibrillation exists. The atria do not contract but merely fibrillate. The ventricular response is irregular with only a portion of the atrial impulses being transmitted to the ventricle. The ventricular rate is usually rapid in untreated cases. The ECG tracing will show small fibrillatory waves or no waves of atrial activity at all. The QRS complexes may show minor degrees of distortion associated with abnormal ventricular excitation (Fig. 147).

NODAL RHYTHMS

Nodal Premature Contractions. Any impulse originating from the AV node of necessity causes retrograde atrial excitation. This creates a P vector directed away from the AV node and toward the right shoulder. A PR interval of less than .10 second with a P vector compatible with a nodal focus is called a nodal impulse.

When an impulse originating from the node creates a premature contraction it is called a nodal premature contraction. These have been separated into three distinct groups: upper, middle, and lower nodal impulses. Upper nodal impulses have a nodal type P vector with the P wave just preceding the QRS complex. It is thought that an impulse originating high in the node will cause atrial excitation before the ventricle is stimulated. Middle nodal impulses are those with no visible P wave. The atrial events occur simultaneously with ventricular excitation and are lost. Lower nodal impulses allow the ventricle to be stimulated before atrial excitation. The QRS complex is followed by a P wave which behaves like a nodal type P wave (Fig. 148).

Nodal prematurities are followed by a com-

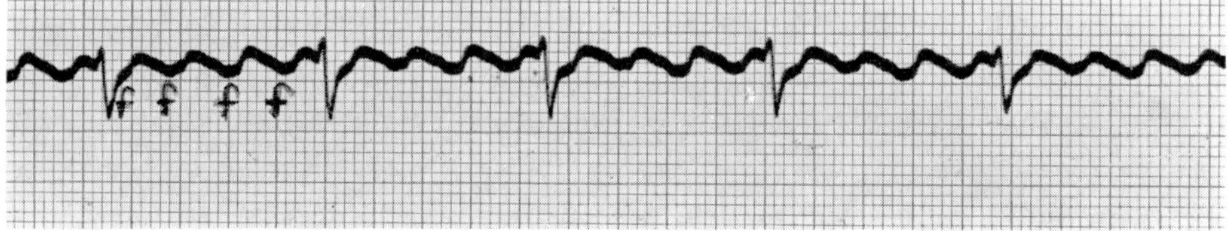

Figure 146. Atrial flutter as seen in Lead III.

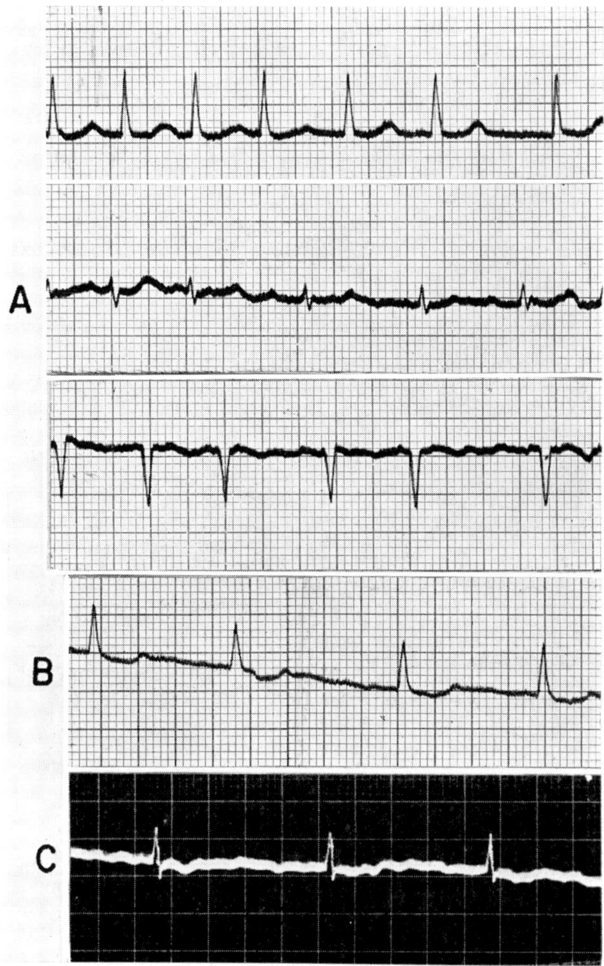

Figure 147. A) Rapid atrial fibrillation. B) After digitalization. C) So called flutter-fibrillation.

pensatory pause since the SA node discharges at its usual time and one SA impulse is lost (Fig. 149). The QRS complex is usually normal. If the impulse originates low enough in the node it may be originating just from one main bundle and resemble a bundle branch block complex.

Nodal Rhythm. When the pacemaker for the heart becomes the AV node, it is called nodal rhythm. The rate is slow, approximately 50 per minute, and regular. The AV node characteristically is slower than the SA node. The impulses look like the nodal impulses described above, but are constant and comprise the basic rhythm. Nodal rhythm may be either upper, middle or lower nodal in origin (Fig. 150).

Nodal Tachycardia. Whenever the AV node emits impulses more rapidly than the SA node, it becomes the cardiac pacemaker. When this rate exceeds 100 a minute, it is a nodal tachycardia. Like atrial tachycardia, it may occur in paroxysms with a sudden onset and sudden termination. Often the two conditions are clinically indistinguishable.

Nodal Escape. If a period of sinus arrest occurs, a lower cardiac center usually takes over the job of pacemaker. The AV node is the next highest center and it may initiate the impulse. This is called nodal escape. The impulse has the usual characteristics of a nodal impulse. It differs from a nodal prematurity in that it follows a long pause or period of arrest and the prematurity occurs early. The impulse may de-

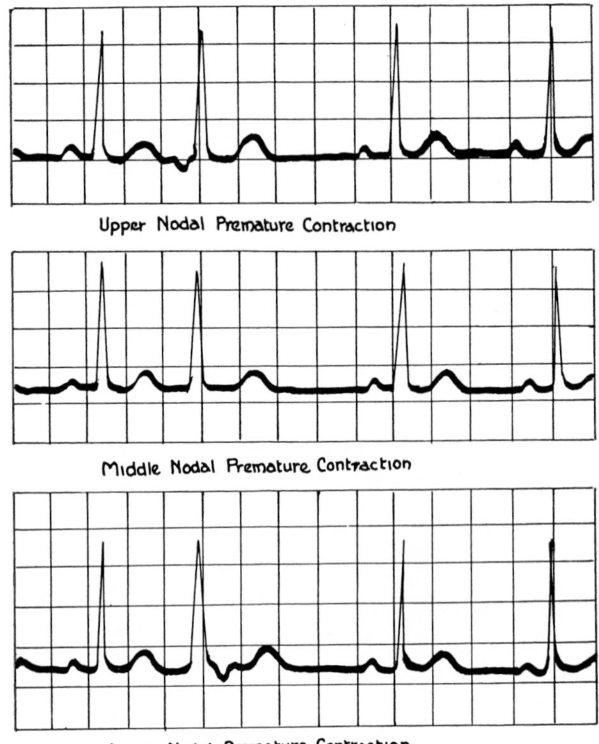

Figure 148.

Figure 149. Nodal premature contractions.

scend farther down the AV node to either bundle and finally descend to the ventricular muscle, or the heart may cause excitation entirely. The gradual depression of the focus of origin is very important clinically as it heralds the onset of cardiac arrest and is an emergency consideration.

Accelerated Nodal Conduction. (See Chapter X).

VENTRICULAR RHYTHMS

Ventricular Prematurities. When an impulse originates prematurely from the ventricle it is called a ventricular premature contraction. The impulse occurs early and is followed by a compensatory pause. The focus initiates ventricular excitation in only one ventricle. Thus the septum is activated only from one surface (Figs. 151 and 152). The time for excitation is prolonged and the magnitude of the resultant vector is increased. This causes increased QRS duration, to .12 sec. or more, and marked increase in the size of the QRS complex.

Ventricular Tachycardia. When tachycardia is the result of a ventricular pacemaker it is called ventricular tachycardia. The rate is usually between 150 and 250 per minute. Ventricular tachycardia is initiated by a ventricular prematurity and may be preceded by several prematurities just prior to onset. The rate may not be entirely regular and the cycle length may vary as much as .04 sec. The QRS complexes are widened to .12 sec. or more. The P waves are slower and are at an independent rate.

The demonstration of the P waves is often absolutely necessary to establish a diagnosis, due to the frequency of widened QRS complexes with those tachycardias having aberrant conduction (early ventricular excitation). Even a sinus tachycardia may be confused with ventricular tachycardia if the P waves are not

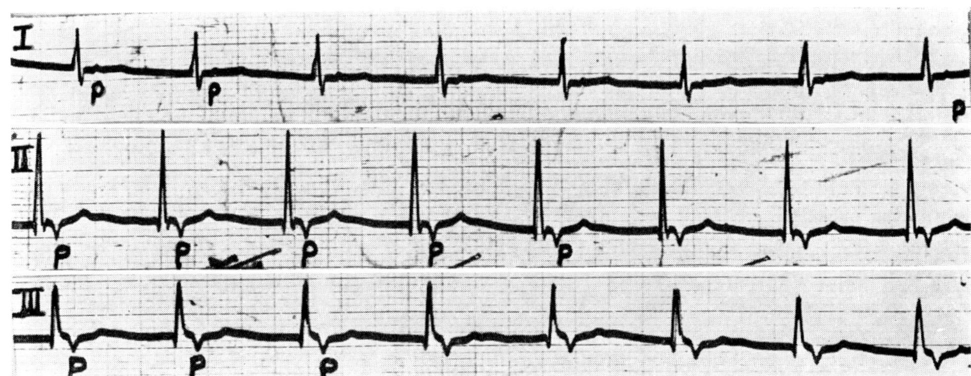

Figure 150. Nodal rhythm.

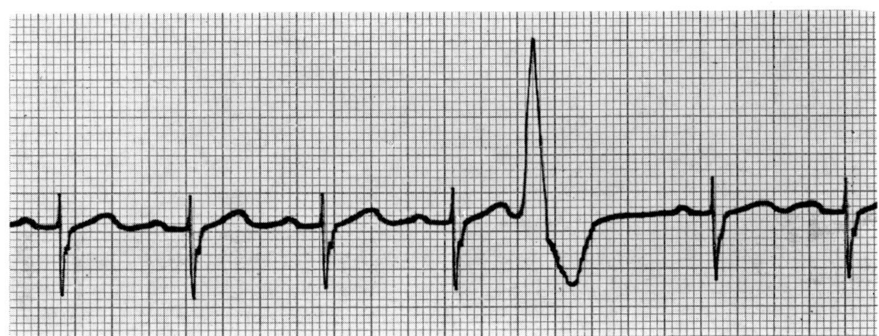

Figure 151. A simple ventricular premature contraction.

found. Occasionally special leads, including esophageal leads, will be necessary to establish the presence of P waves.

Ventricular impulses from other foci may be interspersed throughout the record. Two foci may alternate, thus producing a bi-directional ventricular tachycardia. This is most often seen as a complication of digitalis intoxication. Termination of the tachycardia is followed by a full compensatory pause (Fig. 153).

Ventricular Fibrillation. Ventricular tachycardia may progress into ventricular fibrillation. The ventricles cease to contract and merely fibrillate at a rate between 130 and 500. The ventricular complexes may appear as fairly uniform oscillations of eight to ten millimeters' amplitude and then gradually decay with subsequent hypoxia. Terminally the oscillations appear as low amplitude undulations.

The atria continue to beat independently until hypoxia develops.

Recovery from ventricular fibrillation has been known to occur after a period of five minutes. It is nevertheless a serious emergency and is frequently death dealing.

AV BLOCK

First Degree AV Block. When transmission through the AV conduction system is unduly prolonged it is called an AV block. If the delay results only in prolongation of the PR interval it is called a first degree AV block (Fig. 154).

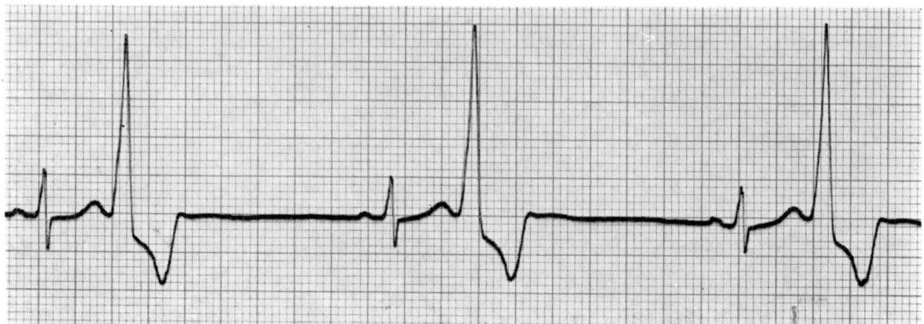

Figure 152. Ventricular premature contractions producing bigeminy.

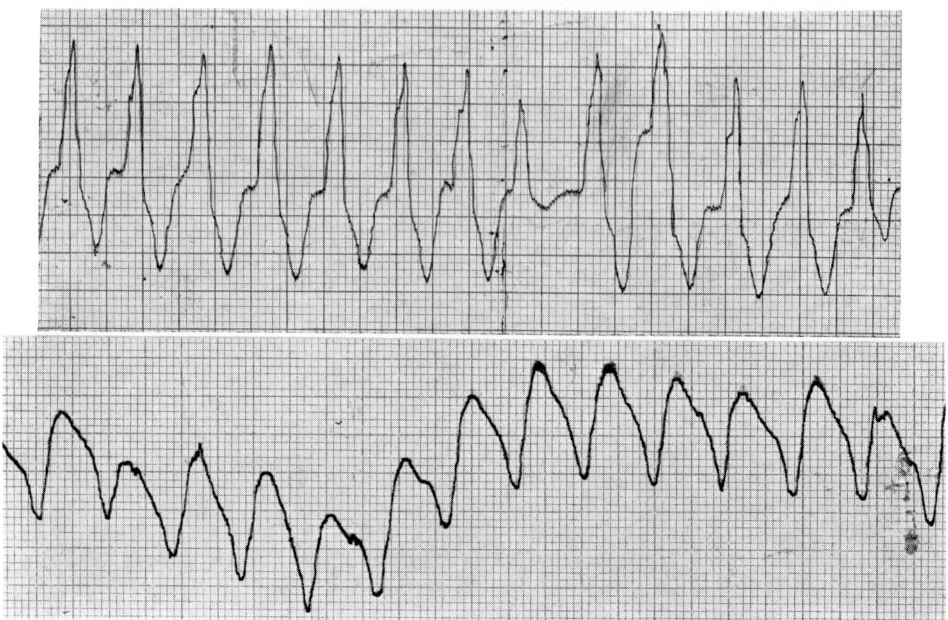

Figure 153. Two examples of ventricular tachycardia.

Second Degree AV Block. The delay may be great enough to prevent the transmission of the impulse part of the time. This results in a P wave without a following QRS complex. This is called a second degree AV block (Fig. 155). When this occurs with progressive prolongation of the PR interval until a QRS complex is lost, it is called a Wenckebach phenomenon (Fig. 156).

Complete AV Block. The inhibition at the AV node may be great enough to prevent the transmission of atrial impulses altogether. In this instance the atria beat independent of the ventricles. This situation is called a third degree AV block, or complete AV dissociation (Fig. 157). The ventricular impulse may be initiated by a lower focus in the node, in which case the ventricular complexes will appear normal; or the impulse may originate in the ventricle with a wide QRS complex of a ventricular focus. In the latter instance the ventricular rate is commonly slower and it is called an idioventricular response.

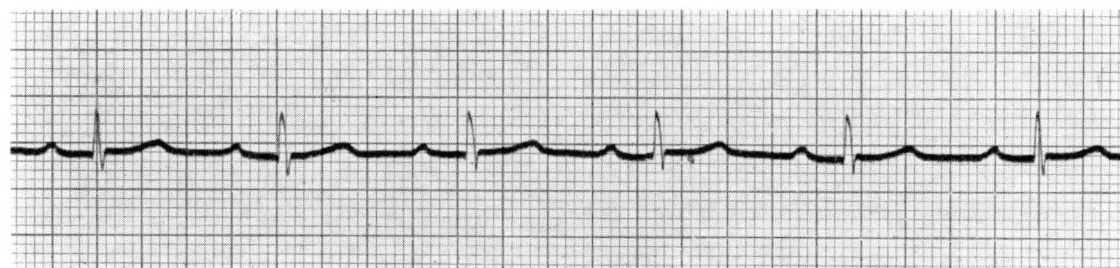

Figure 154. 1st degree AV block.

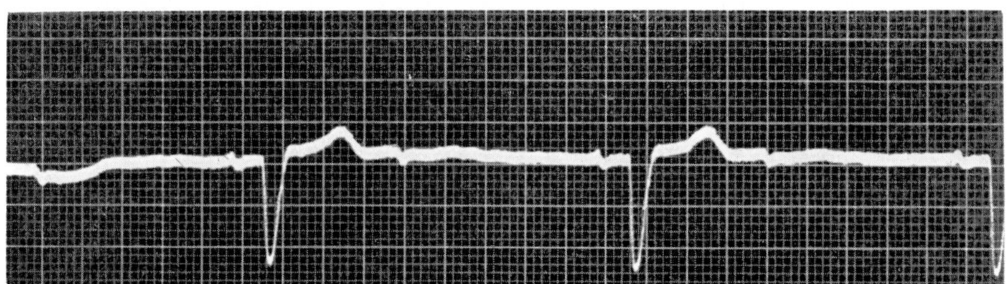

Figure 155. 2nd degree AV block.

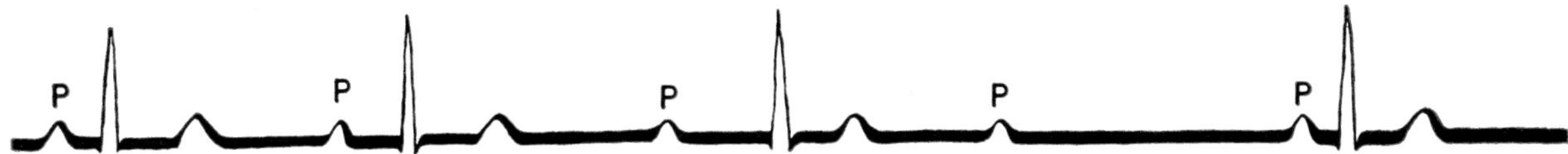

Figure 156. Wenkebach's phenomenon.

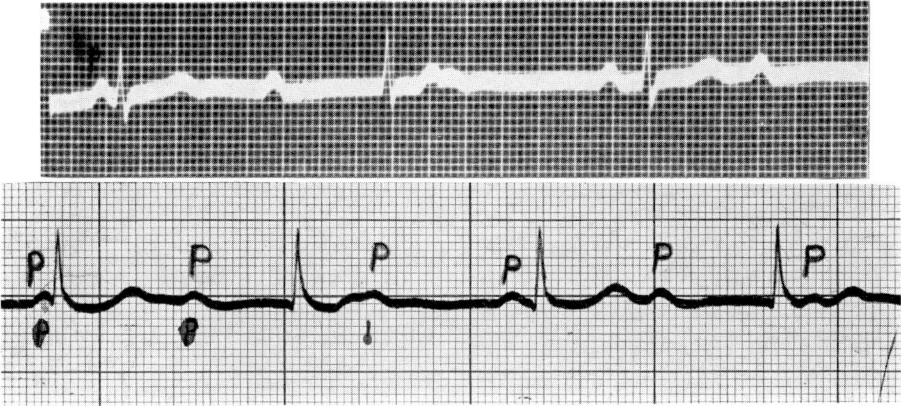

Figure 157. Two examples of complete AV block.

XV

The Interpretation

THE ELECTROCARDIOGRAPHIC interpretation should be made in such a way as to give a maximum amount of information and a minimum amount of confusion. Dogmatic interpretations must be avoided as there are too many variables in the ECG. The maximum benefit of the tracing can only be obtained by clinical correlation.

The value of comparative records cannot be over emphasized. An inverted T3 may be a normal finding in one individual and an important change indicating disease in still another. Only adequate base line records will resolve the question on certain occasions.

The first part of the interpretation is entirely descriptive. One notes the basic rhythm, e.g., normal sinus rhythm rate 75 per minute. Secondary arrhythmias are noted, such as normal sinus rhythm with occasional ventricular premature contractions. Any of the numerous arrhythmias may be present or combinations of arrhythmias, e.g., complete AV block with sinus arrhythmia (sinus arrhythmia is noted in the P waves).

The intervals are described: PR interval, QRS duration, QT interval. The character of the P waves may be described as normal, increased amplitude or duration, or abnormal characteristic, notching or abnormally directed P vector. The QRS complex is described in terms of amplitude and configuration, e.g., S_1 S_2 S_3, .04 sec. Q wave in Lead III and Lead II, R R′ at V1. The ST segments are noted to be isoelectric, elevated or depressed. The T wave configuration may be described as normal, peaked, increased amplitude, or low amplitude. The presence of U waves is noted.

The mean QRS axis is determined in the frontal plane in degrees and the transition noted in the V leads. This describes its spatial orientation. The T vector is described in axis degrees for the frontal plane and its transition in the V leads. From this information the spatial mean QRS-T angle can be estimated from the spatial angle chart.

A simple descriptive interpretation is not much help to the clinician and requires no great skill. He wants to know whether the record is normal or abnormal and if possible what the abnormality means. This phase of the reading is the clinical interpretation. If the record is normal by the above measurements, one should state, "*the record is within normal limits.*" Any arrhythmia should be noted also in this portion of the reading.

If the PR interval was noted to be abnormally prolonged for the rate and age, one states, "first degree AV block," or other AV conduction disturbances are noted such as second degree AV block or complete AV block.

A prolonged QRS duration is interpreted in the clinical section as left bundle branch block, right bundle branch block, intraventricular conduction defect, accelerated nodal conduction (WPW), S_1 S_2 S_3 pattern a normal variant, or delay in activation over the right ventricle usually a normal variant. It is good to point out than an ominous sounding term (S_1 S_2 S_3) is a normal variant and not worry the attending physician with trivial information.

If the QT interval was found to be abnormally prolonged, it should be mentioned in the clinical interpretation as "prolonged QT interval consistent with . . . ." Electrolyte disturbance and rheumatic carditis are both frequent causes. Often the attending physician will have asked for the tracing to detect changes consistent with some specific problem such as hypopotassemia.

Abnormally large P waves should be cited as consistent with atrial enlargement or dilatation. Don't try to distinguish between left and right atrial enlargement on the electrocardiogram alone. You will be wrong as often as right and it is better taste to give less information and be right when you give it.

When right axis deviation and precordial leads suggest its presence, one should say, "right axis deviation consistent with right ventricular hypertrophy," or "right axis deviation with R R′ at V1 consistent with right ventricular enlargement or right bundle branch block."

As there are many causes for a wide spatial mean QRS-T angle, it is probably best to note it as just an abnormality unless other changes accompany it. T wave changes, after all, can mean anything from myocardial infarction to changes secondary to a recent carbohydrate intake. Dogmatic interpretations without knowledge of the case do more harm than good. Serial electrocardiograms are very helpful in evaluating T wave abnormalities.

When a combination of findings suggesting left ventricular hypertrophy is present, it is probably safe to make the interpretation, "abnormal record with increased QRS amplitude. Widened QRS-T angle and ST segment changes, consistent with left ventricular hypertrophy."

ST segment changes that do not appear normal should be noted, e.g., "ST segment changes consistent with epicardial injury. Suggest serial records for evaluation."

Classic infarctions may be diagnosed. Digitalis may be suspected. There are many valuable interpretations that can be made. One should never forget that an electrocardiogram does have limitations. It is used best with clinical information, previous comparative records and, in some cases, serial records. Because the electrocardiogram is often credited with infallibility by the uninitiated, avoid at all times dogmatic interpretations from the electrocardiogram alone.

There is still much valuable information to be learned from the use of the electrocardiogram. As yet we have only scratched the surface with its application. Even so, it is already a routine diagnostic procedure for both cardiac and general internal medicine problems.

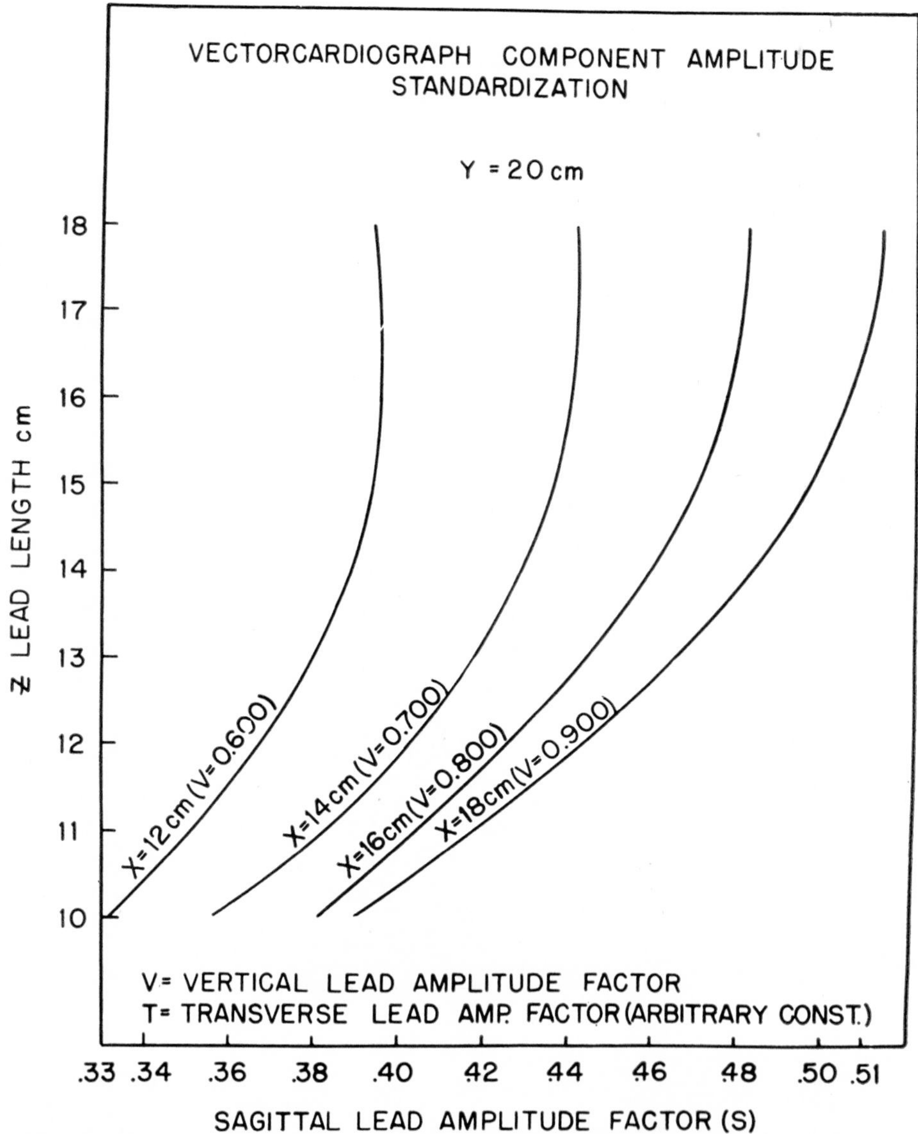

Figure 158. The amplification or standardization for the three vectorcardiographic leads (X, Y, Z) can be determined by, 1) selecting the chart with the proper Y lead length, 2) placing a straight edge at the left hand margin at the measured length of the Z lead, 3) noting the point where the straight edge intersects the line representing the correct X lead lngth and 4) reading the amplification for Z (sagittal lead) directly beneath the point of intersection. The X amplification is given on the same curved line representing the X lead length. The amplification of Y is 1.00.

Given a Y lead of 20 cm. length, a Z lead of 17 cm. length and an X lead of 12 cm. length, the amplifications are read as,

Y = 1.00
X = .60
Z = .40 (approximation).

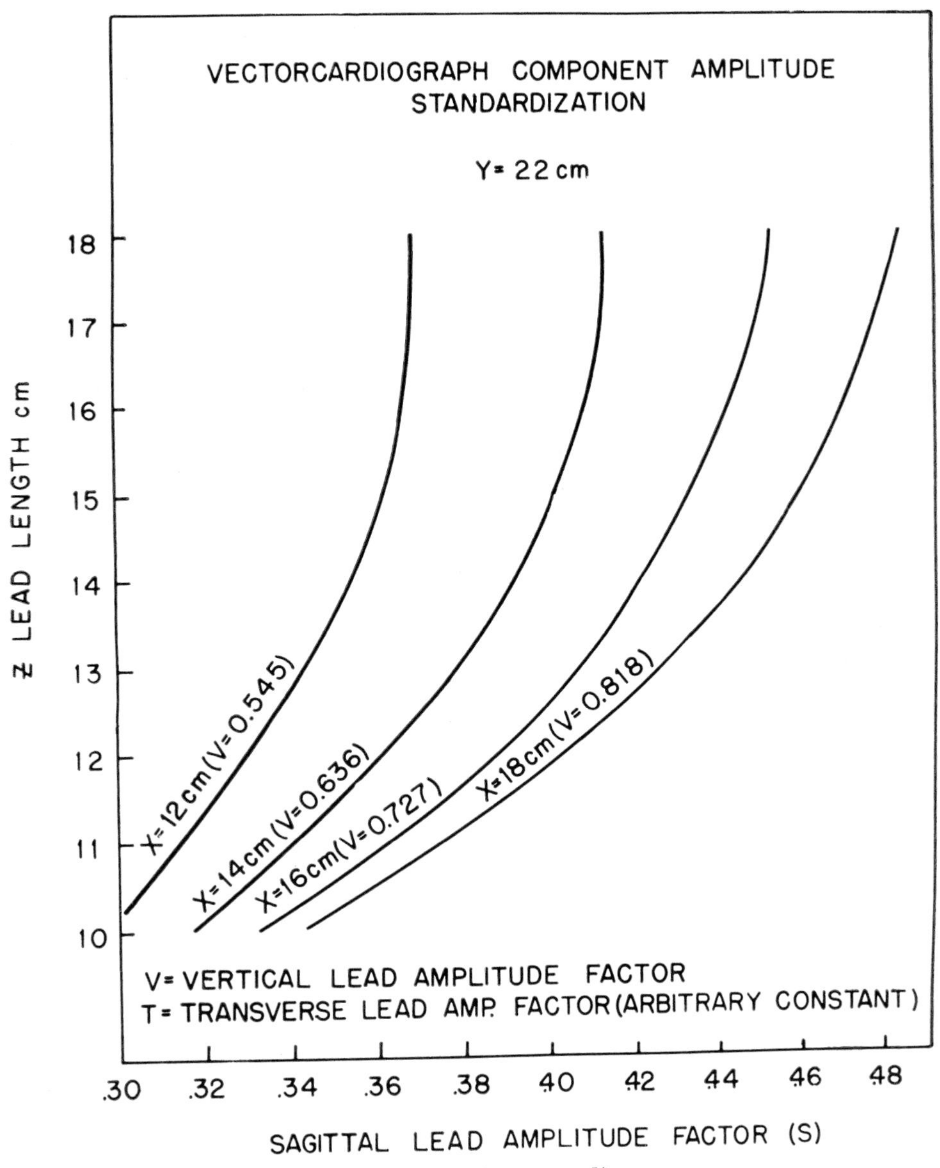

Figure 158 (Continued).

The most common lead lengths used in the adult are, Y = 30 cm., T = 22 cm. and the sagittal varies. In such a case Y = 1.00, T = .73 and sagittal amplification is as follows:

Sagittal Lead 15 cm. = .36 amplification
16 cm. = .38
17 cm. = .40
18 cm. = .41
19 cm. = .42
20 cm. = .43
21 cm. = .44

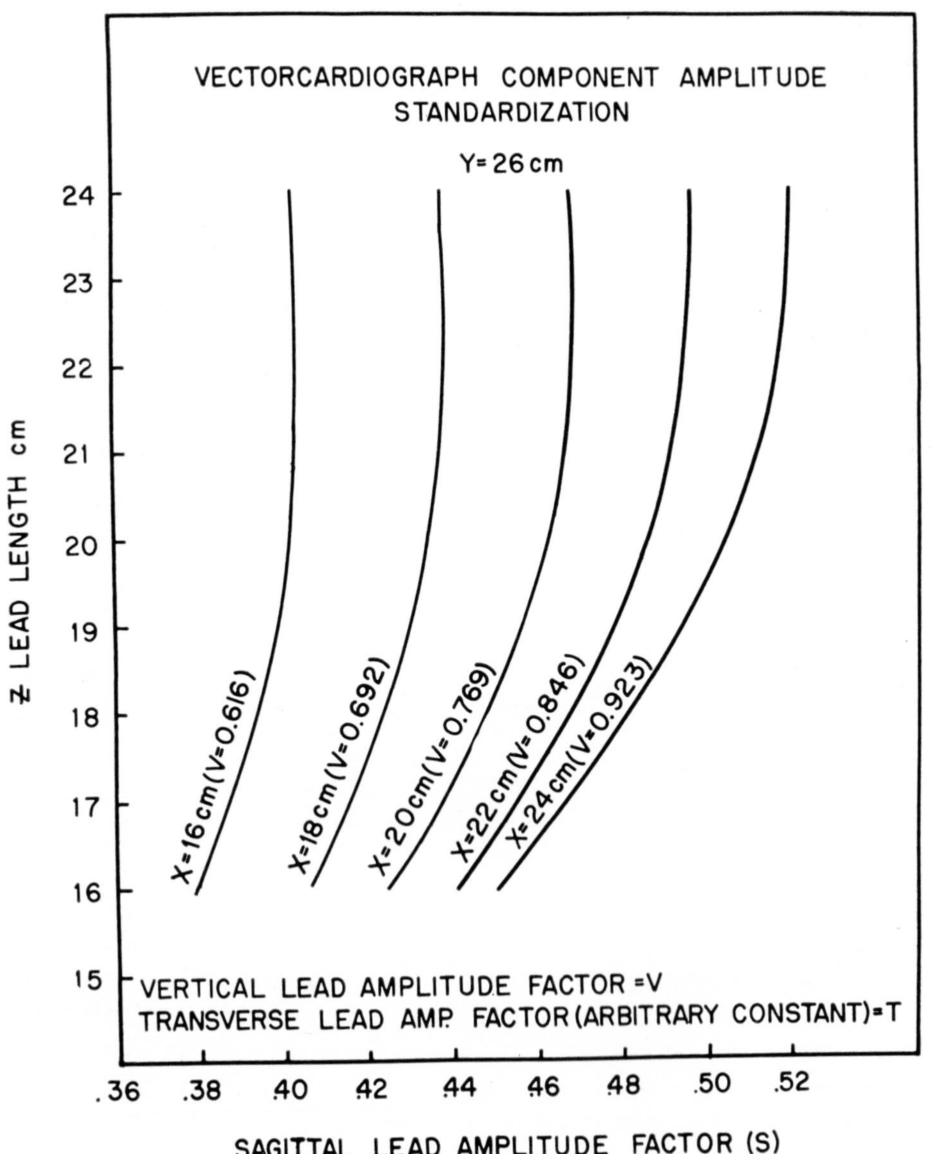

Figure 158 (Continued).

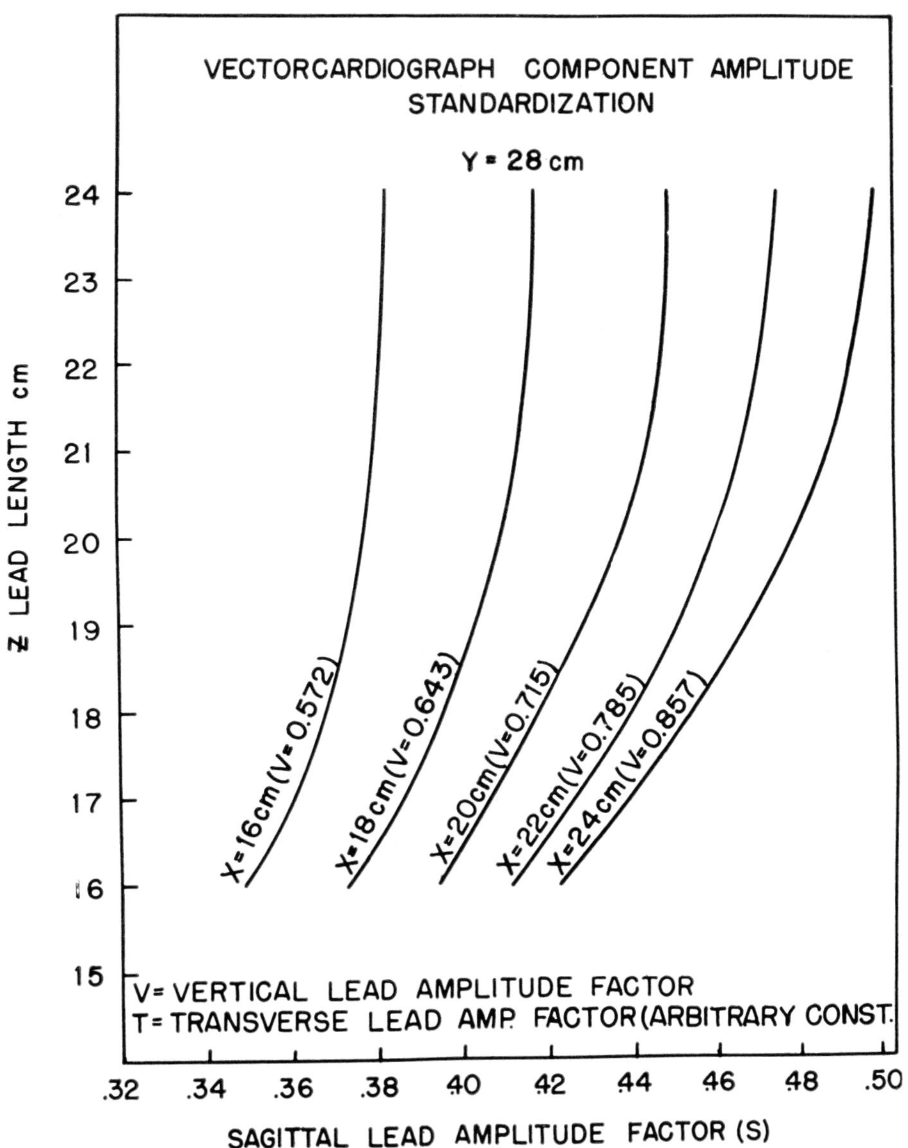

Figure 158 (Continued).

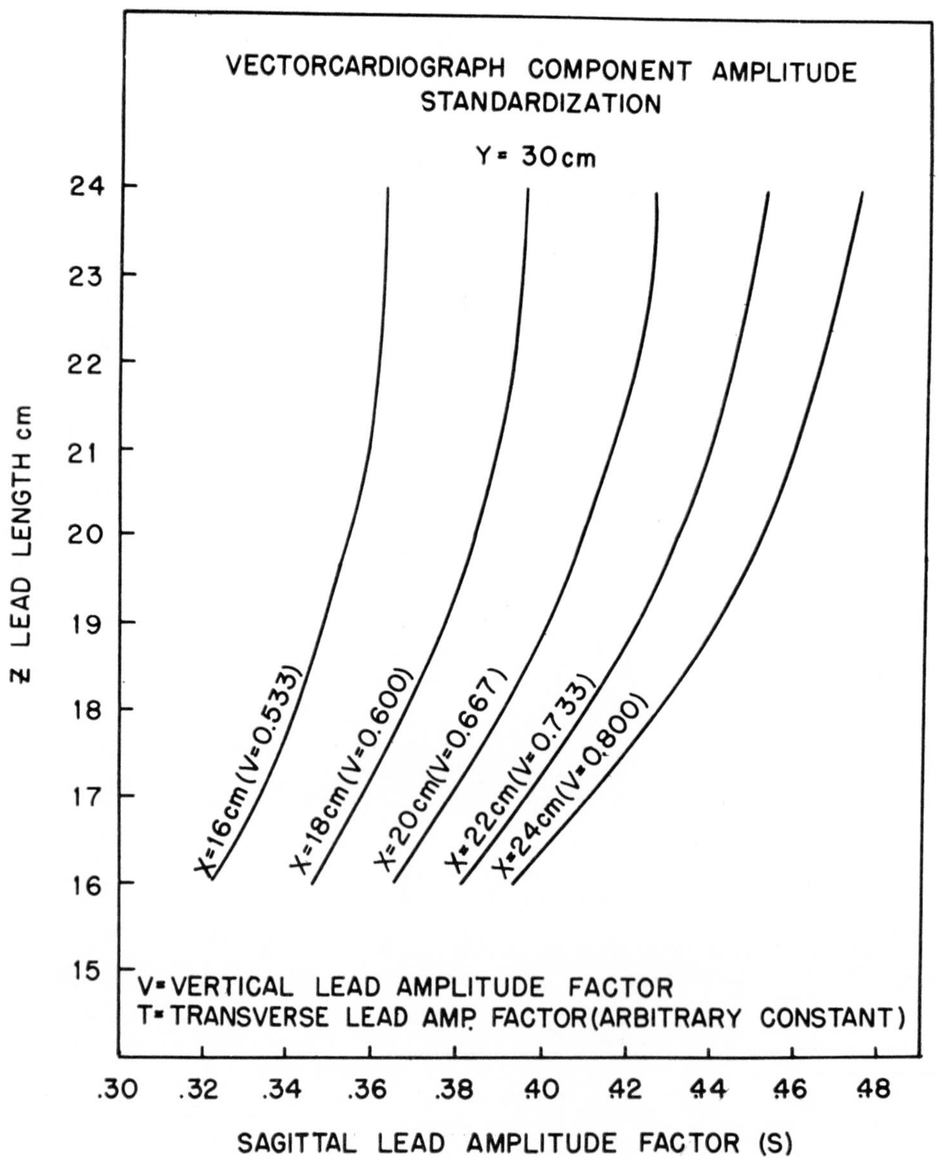

Figure 158 (Continued).

Index

W

Z